Safety in Electromedical Technology

Norbert Leitgeb

Interpharm Press, Inc.
Buffalo Grove, IL

Invitation to Authors

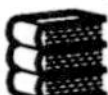 Interpharm Press publishes books focused upon applied technology and regulatory affairs impacting Healthcare Manufacturers worldwide. If you are considering writing or contributing to a book applicable to the pharmaceutical, biotechnology, medical device, diagnostic, cosmetic, or veterinary medicine manufacturing industries, please contact our Director of Publications.

Social Responsibility Programs

Reforestation

 Interpharm Press is concerned about the impact of the worldwide loss of trees upon both the environment and the availability of new drug sources. Therefore, Interpharm supports global reforestation and commits to replant trees sufficient to replace those used to meet the paper needs to print its books.

Pharmakos-2000

 Through its Pharmakos-2000 program, Interpharm Press fosters the teaching of pharmaceutical technology. Under this program, complimentary copies of selected Interpharm titles are regularly sent to every College and School of Pharmacy worldwide. It is hoped that these books will be useful references to faculty and students in advancing the practice of pharmaceutical technology.

Commissioned in the UK by Sue Horwood of Medi-Tech, Publications Limited, Storrington, West Sussex, on behalf of Interpharm Press, Inc., USA. General Scientific Advisor: Robin N. Stephens, Global Regulatory Associates, UK

---

10 9 8 7 6 5 4 3 2 1

ISBN: 1-57491-014-0

Copyright © 1996 by Interpharm Press, Inc. All rights reserved.

Interpharm Press, Inc.
1358 Busch Parkway
Buffalo Grove, IL 60089, USA
Phone: + 1 + 847 + 459-8480
Fax: + 1 + 847 + 459-6644

Contents

Introduction

Today, there is a common opinion that the safety of medical devices is the responsibility of manufacturers and clinical engineers. Unfortunately, people with this opinion do not recognize that the increasing complexity of medical device applications, whether alone or in combination with other medical or nonmedical devices (see "Medical Systems", chapter 5), requires the user's cooperation as well. It is, therefore, not merely a moral imperative that the user not reject his responsibility. In day-to-day medical applications, the importance of technical devices requires that medical staff members have at least a minimum of insight into the potential risks of medical technical devices. They, too, cannot ignore safety rules.

During the last century the increased use of drugs has led to today's undisputed need for basic knowledge in biochemistry and pharmacology. Likewise, at the end of the 20th century, the need for basic knowledge in the safety aspects of technical devices cannot be questioned.

This book is not intended to discuss in detail the numerous safety standards in medical device technology—for three reasons: (1) It is intended to provide a *basis* for understanding safety considerations. (2) Any detailed discussion of standards would exceed the practical limits of this book. As standards are continuously developing, such a discussion would rapidly become obsolete. (3) If the discussion becomes obsolete, there is a risk that the use of standards would be renounced by those who must work with them, such as design or test engineers.

This book is intended to provide basic principles and to discuss the context of safety considerations that should be known by all persons responsible for medical device safety, namely, engineers who design, construct, test, or service medical devices, as well as users who must be aware of specific problems and how to identify, estimate, and handle risk situations properly.

Therefore, chapter 1 addresses general aspects of the identification and individual perception of risks to which we are exposed in daily life. Using an example, essential safety conclusions and strategies are deduced, leading to the three-column concept in medical device technology, which is based on the common responsibility of the manufacturer, the user, and hospital management.

Chapter 2 is devoted to legal aspects. Everyone has a legal claim to rely on care at work. We, too, are obliged to perform our duties with care and conscientiousness. The aim of standardization is to define the reasonable effort that must be undertaken by the involved parties, as well as the requirements that must be met by medical devices.

Supported by practical examples, chapter 3 shows that the most important safety risks related to the application of electromedical devices are derived from basic electrotechnical relations.

The biological effects of electricity are discussed in chapter 4. It shows that current is responsible for the consequences of an accident. From electrical current's bioeffects, safety limits are deduced and protective precautions in medical device technology are derived.

The safety aspects of electromedical devices—the resulting safety concept, risk analysis and assessment, and visual external safety inspection are discussed at the beginning of chapter 5. The section on internal safety inspection describes critical points that may still be found in many newly developed devices. This should give hints to design engineers to help them avoid weak points, and support test engineers in finding them. Finally, there is a discussion of safety problems that might occur if medical devices and non-medical devices are connected to complex medical systems, such as electrophysiological devices connected to commercial PCs.

Chapter 6 takes into account that medical devices, in particular, might include or be exposed to additional risk factors, such as liquids, burn-promoting gases, or explosive mixtures. An examination of the device-related aspects of infections and their prevention conclude this chapter.

The last chapter contains the basic strategies of the electric power supply in hospitals, the hierarchical concept, and the means by which it is assured that, at a minimum, life-supporting devices remain supplied with electrical energy.

This book should help open eyes to safety risks, and, by providing knowledge about them, help to avoid danger and meet safety requirements, to the benefit of both patients and personnel.

Norbert Leitgeb
Graz, Austria, 1996

1 Risk and Safety

For the pessimist death begins with birth; for the optimist death occurs only at the end of life. Regardless, it is a fact that we are continuously exposed to risks. However, our risk perception is influenced by a variety of factors, and we individually estimate risk quite differently. In his play *Lumpazivagabundus*, Nestroy, the famous Austrian author, lets one of his actors, the shoemaker Knieriem, explain why he does not want to settle down and have a family: He is convinced that a comet will strike the earth soon and destroy it. Although the collision of a comet with the earth is an extremely improbable event, for Knieriem this possibility poses an overwhelming threat.

This chapter shows that where we do not have enough experience to have developed good judgment, our perception of risks and, as a consequence, our awareness of problems depends on several additional factors. We must accept that, in principle, total safety does not exist, and anything that can go wrong will, in fact, go wrong. Therefore, the statement that something is safe just because nothing has happened is not convincing. However, although an accident may be caused by a single factor, it can also be avoided by removing only a single risk factor from the causal chain.

1.1 Risk Perception

In common speech the term *risk,* as in "the risk of being fined because of illegal parking", is frequently used to mean the "probability of occurrence of an event". In safety considerations "risk" covers even more than that: It also includes the consequences of an event. Specifically, risk is understood to be the product of the probability of occurrence and the degree of severity of harm.

risk = probability of occurrence × damage

In medical device technology this is taken into account by classifying risks into different groups (see "Device Risk Groups" later in this chapter). However, there are risks other than those inherent in medical devices in health care. Additional hazards can arise from the use of or the presence of flammable or even explosive substances (disinfectants, anaesthetic gases), dangerous radiation (lasers, X-rays, radioactivity), radioactive substances, and infectious germs.

With the given formula, risk can be estimated, but it is in the nature of things that the result cannot, of course, be more than an estimate. For a given observation period, risk estimation is more inaccurate the less frequently an event occurs, meaning that less specific experience is available. Nuclear power plants are illustrative examples. Initially, the risk of a worst-case scenario, the largest assumable accident, was estimated. Later, another estimate for a "super–worst-case scenario" became necessary, which demonstrates an interesting fact for linguists; namely, bad → worse → worst can be further enhanced by the term *super-worst.*

In spite of all the attempts to quantify risk, the results influence an individual's estimation of it and one's behavior while handling risky things to only a minor degree. Do you travel by train just because you know that the risk of accidents is significantly lower compared with traveling by car?

The reason for an individual's distorted view lies in the subjective perception of risk, which depends on a variety of additional factors. Today, the importance and consequences of risk are investigated scientifically. There are many parameters to how we perceive risk. For example, in traveling in a car, the risk is perceived to be smaller than it really is. We are *familiar* with its use; we are convinced that we can *manage the risk by our own efforts* (e.g., by adequate behaviour, rapid reaction, and the use of safety belts or airbags). In fact, the skill involved in driving a car seems to be one of the most fairly distributed abilities on earth: One rarely finds anyone who claims to be a bad driver! Further calming factors are that the individual derives *personal benefit* from driving, and becomes *accustomed* to daily reports of car accidents that have a *lower catastrophic potential* in contrast to accidents involving a large number of people (e.g., airplane crashes or ferry accidents) that receive a large amount of media attention.

In the case of the diffuse fear of electric and magnetic fields from high tension power lines (Leitgeb 1990), the situation is quite different: Although *risks could not* (yet) *be proven* and estimates were based on *uncertain hypothetical assumptions*, they often were overestimated by the general population. This has been additionally supported by the lack of *common knowledge* of physics; periodically increased *media attention* in combination with sales promotions for various protective devices and corrective actions; the *lack of trust* in authorities who are publishing low risk estimates in an effort to calm the public; the *small possibility of influencing* or avoiding electromagnetic fields *by one's own means;* the generally *unclear individual benefit* (Why high tension lines? My current comes out of my mains socket outlet!); and, finally, the fact that this risk is *man made* in that it stems from technical sources rather than being an effect of natural sources that must be accepted.

The same risk factor, electric and magnetic fields, can be perceived quite differently and even considered to be negligible if it is produced by one's own electrical appliances. This occurs in spite of the fact that the fields may be considerably higher than those associated with high tension lines. Only at first glance does this seem to be a contradiction. The reason for the low risk perception is caused by the *awareness* of the evident *individual benefit* and the feeling that one is *able to switch off* the field source at any time.

Research shows that people's perception of risk, independent of their education, is subject to these distorting influences. Table 1.1 summarizes the most important factors that influence individual risk perception and the resulting awareness of safety problems. To get a feeling for the problems in medical technology, a very important strategy is to enhance one's knowledge of risks and to learn to identify risk factors.

1.2 Life's Daily Pitfalls

Did anything go wrong today? Did you forget something or miss an appointment because you were stuck in a traffic jam? Did you miss the bus by an inch, or did your shoelace tear when you were already in a hurry?

Cofactors	Risk Perception	
	High	Low
Objective risk	large	small
Risk estimation	uncertain, unreliable	certain, reliable
Risk factor	unfamiliar	familiar
Personal benefit	unclear, small	clear, large
Personal control	small	high
Personal decision range	small	large
Familiarity	low	high
Own knowledge	small	large
Media attention	large	small
Consequences	unknown, delayed, feared	known acute, unfeared
Children at risk	yes	no
Risk source	technical	natural

Table 1.1. Parameters of Risk Perception

These examples illustrate that we are exposed to different kinds of risks continuously. Fortunately, as a rule, we succeed in handling them because we have developed our own strategies to reduce risks. In most cases we rely on redundancy, that is, the availability of a second equivalent alternative that might be used if the first fails. In addition, we assume that any mistake will not activate other existing risk factors.

For instance, if it is very important for you to get up on time because you would otherwise miss your plane for your vacation, you probably will not rely only on your own alarm clock, but will use a second one (redundant safety precaution), or perhaps ask someone to give you a call (second redundant safety precaution), assuming that it would be unlikely that both of you would oversleep at the same time. In safety terms you rely on the decoupling of existing risk factors. But in spite of all precautions, it can happen that something will go wrong and you will get into trouble anyway.

This can be explained by a further example (adapted from Perrow 1984). Imagine that in the evening your parents came to discuss how they would look after your apartment during your vacation. You were still upset from a quarrel with your neighbor, caused by the persistent barking of his dog which, together with the continuous noise from a nearby building site, had made you lose your temper. Afterward, you and your wife decided to watch the night thriller about a jail breakout before going to sleep. Because you were invited to a job interview the following day, you had planned to sleep longer. Thus, you handed your alarm clock over to your wife, asking her to wake you up in the morning before leaving.

However, because of the night thriller (first risk factor), your wife went to sleep later than usual. In addition, awaking to the alarm clock is unfamiliar (second risk factor), resulting in oversleeping. Being cautious, you had asked your parents to call you in the morning; therefore, you were still able to get up in time (this redundant safety means proved to be useful). Because your wife was late, there was no time to prepare breakfast (risk factor), and she had to borrow a neighbour's car (further risk factor) to reach the office in time.

Unfortunately, especially in the morning, coffee is very important to you. Therefore, you decide to have at least instant coffee and take the time to heat some water. But when it is ready, you realize that the instant coffee had been used up by your visitors the evening before (this shows an unexpected coupling with the usually independent event of the visit). Because of the time loss and the missing coffee, you become nervous (risk factor). To make an impression at the interview, you decide to change your suit (next risk factor) and dress in a hurry. Unfortunately, your shoelace tears, which further increases your nervousness (a loose coupling with the time loss). You rush out of your home, and the door shuts. At the car you become aware of leaving the car keys in the suit you wore yesterday. At first, you are not worried because for such cases you have a reserve key hidden in the window box (first redundancy); but then you remember that you had given all the keys to your parents in view of their planned visits during your vacation. Now you are unable to drive your own car (so another unexpected coupling with an independent event has invalidated your safety means). On any other day, you could have used your neighbour's car (second redundancy), but today your wife has taken advantage of that (here we find an event closely coupled with your wife's oversleeping; in safety terms, a consecutive effect). In general you could ask for the other neighbour's car (third redundancy), but because of the recent quarrel with him, this is impossible (further unexpected coupling).

But you are still optimistic, and you decide to take the bus (fourth redundancy). At the bus stop you realize that public transport is on strike because of wage negotiations (further unexpected coupling). When you try to call a taxi (fifth redundancy), you are informed that because of the strike all taxis are in use; thus, the wait would be too long (in safety terms, an aftereffect of the strike). As a last resort, you decide to reach your destination by hitchhiking (sixth redundancy). Unfortunately, you do not succeed. In the nearby jail prisoners successfully have implemented the trick shown on the night thriller and escaped from jail. Therefore, people have been warned not to give a lift to any unknown person (further unexpected coupling). When you finally realize you cannot keep your appointment, you at least want to apologize by phone. To your surprise, however, you find out that a bulldozer at the nearby building site has damaged the telephone cable (further coupling with an independent event). This makes your personal catastrophe unavoidable: Because of a loss of trust in your reliability, you have lost your chance for this job (see Figure 1.1).

1.2.1 Safety Conclusions

This example shows that in spite of multiple safety precautions, accidents may happen. In fact, forgetting the car keys would not have been a problem if your wife had not overslept or if your quarrel with the neighbour had not taken place. Even all these things would have been insignificant if today was not so important. This example also shows that decoupled events may interact, and unexpected or even unforseeable links may be generated. This leads to an important conclusion: Total safety does not exist. Safety precautions can reduce but not fully eliminate risk. In our example even sixfold redundancy was not able to prevent harm.

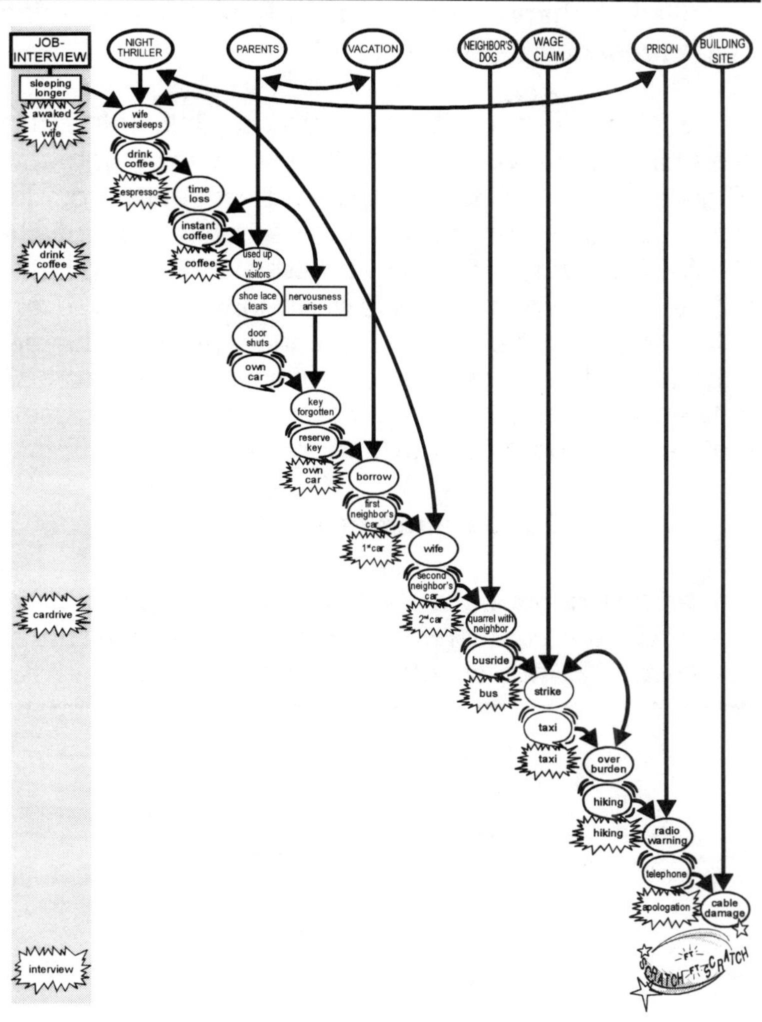

Figure 1.1. Schematic of unexpected couplings of events.

Total safety does not exist!

Safety, however, must be paid for by higher costs or increased time, such as at airports where extra time is required for passenger checks. It may require more inconvenient handling (e.g., use of protective clothing in the presence of toxic agents).

At low safety levels, with comparatively little effort, it is possible to achieve considerable safety improvements (Figure 1.2). For a further increase of safety, cost increases linearly; afterward, it increases exponentially. Finally, at high safety levels even small additional safety improvements involve enormous costs. In every field, including the medical technology field, the accepted safety level is the result of a social compromise between cost and benefit. This leads to the conclusion that safety cannot be provided free of charge:

Safety must be paid for!

On the one hand, because the price must be paid immediately, the cost is well known. On the other hand, the benefit is not so obvious because it lies in the

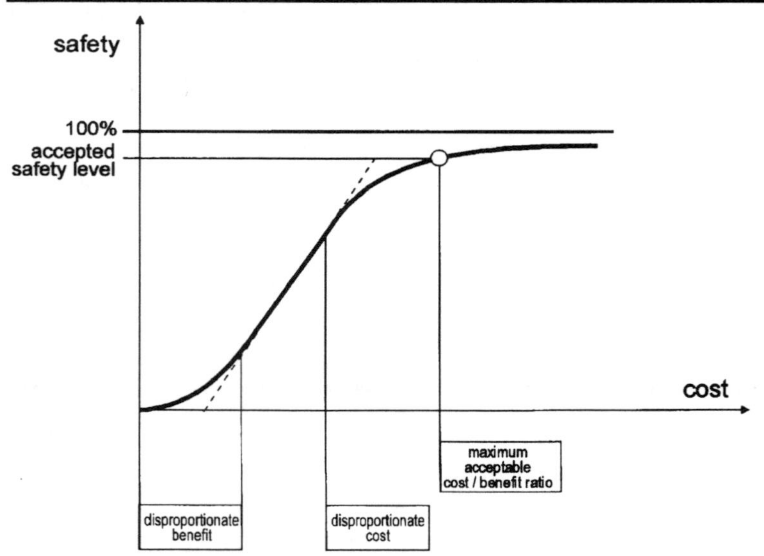

Figure 1.2. Dependence of safety on cost.

nature of prevention that things do not happen. Therefore, safety-related efforts are questioned frequently. One important aspect of safety strategies is to keep people informed and to motivate them to stay cautious and not to wait to learn by harm.

1.3 Safety Strategies

Safety strategy in electrotechnology is based on the assumption that the simultaneous occurrence of two independent failures has such a low probability that prevention of it would not be justifiable economically. As a general rule, electrical devices are designed to provide (only) double (not three-, four- or fivefold) protection. This means that at least a second equivalent protection means must be available (redundancy) to still provide full protection even if the first one fails. It is permitted, however, that a device may be damaged if a first failure occurs, provided that the breakdown itself is not combined with any hazard (as would be the case for infusion pumps, defibrillators, or heart-lung machines).

**Electrical devices provide (only)
double protection!**

The fact that despite all the many precautions, the job interview was missed, demonstrates Murphy's law, which states that everything that can go wrong sometimes will go wrong.

**Everything that can go wrong
sometimes will go wrong!**

If manufacturers are asked to redesign their devices according to the requirements of safety standards, many will argue that it is not necessary because *nothing has ever happened!* It must be stressed that this argument is, of course, no evidence against Murphy's law. Even if the company had a vigilance system without gaps (!), this only would mean that the failure probability is lower than what would be expected, and this, especially for newly developed devices in general, is not notably high. The safety of devices, however, must be assured throughout their whole lifetime, which can be more than 10 years.

A further consequence of our example drawn from daily life is that harm, accidents, or even catastrophes do not have just a single cause; in general, they are the endpoint of a *chain of single events.* Considered separately, none of these events would be critical. But since they happen at the same time, they lead to unexpected or even unpredictable couplings and interactions that may cause something to run out of control and lead to an accident. This can be described by the domino theory: Accidents have no single cause, but are the **endpoints of a chain** of single events!

Accidents never have just a single cause!

This can be explained by a further example, this time in the field of medical device technology: In a hospital a routine check by the user (safety precaution preventive inspection) showed that a defibrillator did not function correctly. A service engineer discovered that the battery was empty. He changed it, made a function check, found it OK, and left. He failed to open the device and make at least a visual internal inspection (see chapter 5).

Two weeks later, the defibrillator was needed for emergency treatment and failed again, this time with fatal consequences: The patient died from heart fibrillation. The result of the investigation was as follows: The injection-molded plastic enclosure of the device, contrary to safety requirements, consisted of two parts that did not sufficiently fit at the storage deepening for electrodes (first risk factor). Obviously, disinfectant liquid had been spilled into the deepening (second risk factor) and had not been wiped out in time (third risk factor), so that it had enough time to enter the device and to accumulate at the bottom. The electronic circuit board had been mounted directly at the bottom without any distance holders (fourth risk factor). In principle, this is not against the requirements, but it allowed the accumulated liquid to connect the soldering points with each other. This caused the battery to discharge. If the service engineer had opened the device, he would have noticed this; however, he did not make an internal visual inspection (fifth risk factor). Obviously, the user inspection intervals were too long (sixth risk factor) to allow detection of this worsening of the device's performance over time.

This shows again that none of the individual events can be identified as the primary reason for the accident. However, this accident could have been avoided if only one of these risk factors had been eliminated (Figure 1.3).

Accidents can be avoided if at least one risk factor in the causal chain is eliminated!

This conclusion provides a very important basis for developing an awareness of safety problems and taking preventive actions. Because the occurrence of an event, as well as its possible interactions and couplings with other risk factors, cannot be foreseen, the

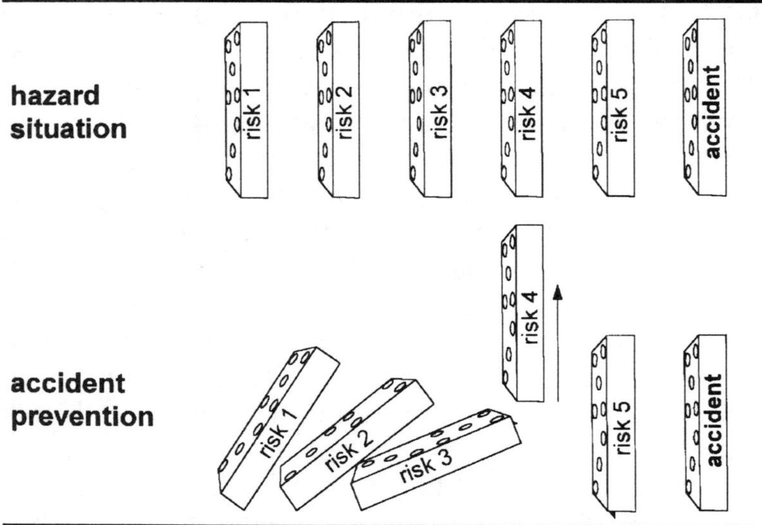

Figure 1.3. Domino theory of accidents.

most important safety strategy is **prevention,** which means not to tolerate any risk, but to eliminate risks as soon as they are identified. Arguments like "nothing will happen" or "nothing happened so far" are safety killers!

Never accept identified risks!

Never rely on safety-killer arguments!

Of course, prevention requires the perception of risk: A child who likes to climb trees and feels safe even on weak and rotten branches obviously is not aware of the risk, which might be obvious to his frightened parents because of their own experience and knowledge of gravity and mechanical strength. Someone who repairs electrical damage in a mains cable with the aid of an (electrically conducting!) adhesive strip behaves like such a child: He lacks an eye for recognizing electrical risks. This demonstrates the importance of a knowledge of technical safety aspects within the high-tech environment that characterizes hospitals today.

Risk identification requires knowledge!

Knowledge of aspects of technical safety is not only necessary for the use of medical devices, but is also required for the design and maintenance of these devices. However, experience shows that design is still dominated by the intended performance of a device. Frequently, safety aspects, even if easy to cover, are considered (too) late or not at all. The cost of eliminating deficiencies, which is often quite small in the design stage, increases exponentially if the product is already produced and on the market. Knowledge of safety technology, therefore, helps to save one's money (and reputation) (Figure 1.4).

1.4 Safety Precautions

We are exposed to risks all the time, even in hospitals. Acknowledging that everything that can go wrong sometimes will go wrong, safety cannot be achieved simply by charging certain groups (e.g., manufacturers or clinical engineers) with the responsibility for safety. This is the main reason why, in the European Union (EU) directive for medical devices as well as in safety standards, it is stated that all parties must take responsibility for technical safety. In particular, the safety concept in medical device technology is based on three assumptions:

1. **The manufacturer** is responsible for the safe design and reliable production of medical devices.

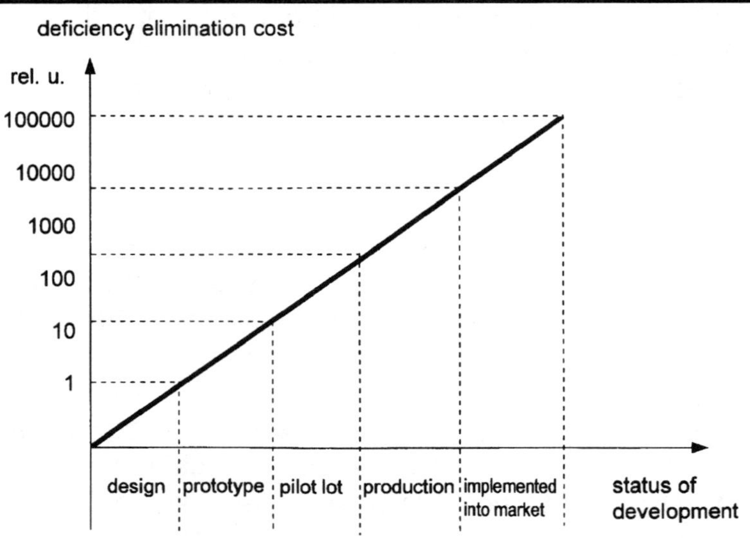

Figure 1.4. Cost of deficiency elimination on device development stage.

2. **The user** must know and follow the conditions and indications for the intended use. He must ascertain proper performance by frequent periodic checks.

3. **Hospital management** must undertake preventive maintenance and periodic safety checks.

Only if all three assumptions are followed can the intended high level of safety be achieved and maintained.

Medical device safety relies on the manufacturer, the user, and hospital management!

1.4.1 Device Safety

There are three ways to provide safety. However, they are not equally efficient and should not be chosen haphazardly.

Unconditional Safety

Unconditional safety is the most effective and should be preferred over all other possibilities. It requires the elimination of risks by design. Of course, it would be possible not to cover devices that contain dangerous electric voltages and just attach the warning *Do not touch!* However, it goes without saying that much more safety is provided by preventing access through adequate insulation. Likewise, it is preferable to prevent a gas bottle from falling by fixing it with a chain, instead of attaching the warning *Do not drop!*

Conflicts may arise if deficiencies are identified by the customer. Then the manufacturer usually proposes a way to solve the problem as cheaply as possible— namely, by attaching a warning instead of changing the design. Standards require that, wherever possible, unconditional safety be preferred. Warnings complement, but do not replace, adequate design.

Conditional Safety

In cases where unconditional safety cannot be realized, it is permitted to apply conditional safety. For example, with X-ray or laser surgical devices, the emission of dangerous radiation cannot be avoided. Risk, however, can be minimized by additional external means, such as limiting access to therapy rooms or by choosing a locking power switch to permit device activation only by authorized (trained) persons. Another possibility is to increase attention (e.g., by demanding more force if the output is to be increased beyond a safe level or to ask for an additional action to activate dangerous outputs). For example, this is commonly required to delete operations on computers or for withdrawing money from a cash station. Further indirect safety means include protective (lead) X-ray skirts, X-ray folding screens, and protective laser glasses.

Descriptive Safety

If conditional safety does not lead to the intended results, the conditions for safe operation must be defined. In general, warnings are used in addition to, rather than instead of, other safety means. Only in cases where it is not possible or appropriate to provide safety by unconditional or conditional means is it permitted to use only descriptive safety, which, for instance, may include requirements for transport, positioning, mounting, connection, operation, replacement, and maintenance ("Handle with care!", "This side up!", "Do not expose to direct sunlight", "Not for explosive zones", "Shake before use!", "Press check button monthly!", or "Exchange filters each year!").

1.4.2 Device Classification

According to the social consensus, to keep costs in a reasonable relation to benefit, the necessary safety efforts are made dependent on the risks inherent to a device (Table 1.2). Depending on their intended use, electrical appliances can be differentiated according to the following safety requirements:

Devices	Design			Electrical Production	Installation	Periodic Inspection		
	double protection	enforced insulation	enforced safety requirements	enforced quality requirements	additional safety means	function	safety parameters	intervals (years)
Group 1 enhanced risk	✔	✔	✔	✔	✔	✔	✔	0.5–2
Group 2 active implants	✔	✔	✔	✔		✔		Determined by physician
Group 3 normal risk	✔	✔			✔	✔	✔	1–3
House-hold	✔							

Table 1.2. Safety Strategies in Electrical Device Technology

- **Household devices:** Used by persons who are conscious and have intact protective reflexes. Used for a short time and under normal environmental conditions. In this case double protection is sufficient. This means that devices must remain safe even in a single-fault condition. However, as it is not possible to rely on special knowledge and increased care by users, special attention must be paid to careless use.

- **Electromedical devices:** Applied to persons who may have reduced reaction ability and/or pain sensation or may be unconscious. Continuous application may be long term and possibly done in the presence of further risk factors, such as oxygen and flammable substances (see chapter 6). This increased hazard potential cannot be managed by device design only. For this reason additional precautions concerning the electrical insulation as well as preventive inspection and maintenance are necessary.

In regard to device technology, electromedical devices must provide double protection. In addition, there are enforced requirements for electrical insulation and separation from mains voltage. Depending on specific hazards, further requirements are defined in special safety standards (e.g., for high frequency surgical devices, laser equipment, and X-ray equipment).

For *electrical installation* it is recommended, and in some countries like Austria and Germany, it is even mandatory, that there be additional safety precautions, such as residual current protective devices in earthed power supply systems that switch off voltage in a single-fault condition, or insulation-monitoring devices in insulated power supply systems that, at a single-fault condition, give an acoustical and visual alarm (see chapters 3 and 7).

The *user* must periodically (daily or weekly) test the performance of critical devices (e.g., the defibrillator output, the charging status of battery-driven devices). In Austria and Germany, for example, hospital management must undertake periodic safety checks of devices already in use. These checks comprise a visual inspection and the measurement of safety parameters. The length of inspection intervals depends on the inherent hazard of a device, ranging from six months to three years. Long intervals indicate, of course, that such inspections are not intended to compete with more frequent performance checks made by a user.

1.4.3 Device Risk Groups

For conformity assessment the EU Medical Device Directive contains a very general classification of all medical devices into four groups, based on their inherent risk, the duration of application, and the site of their biological effect (see chapter 2). Another differentiation has already been established in Austria and Germany: To specify the intervals for periodic inspections, medical devices are classified as follows:

Group 1

Group 1 contains devices with the highest application risk. On the one hand, this can be due to their **principle of operation**—the use of dangerous radiation (laser therapy devices, laser coagulation equipment), dangerous electric currents (nerve and muscle stimulators, electroconvulsive devices, high frequency surgical devices), dangerous voltages (defibrillators, external heart pacemakers), or dangerous temperatures (thermocautery devices, cryosurgical devices).

On the other hand, the enhanced risk can be due to the **function** itself—its critical *accuracy* (infusion pumps, syringe infusion pumps), or its necessary *reliability* (heart-lung machine, lung ventilators, incubators, dialysis equipment, blood filtration devices).

Finally, inherent risk can be caused by the **application site.** Devices or their applied parts that are intended to come into direct contact with the patient's heart (high pressure angiographic injectors, intracardial blood pressure monitors, intracardial electrocardiogram monitors) require special attention. The reason is that our heart is very sensitive to fibrillation by electrical leakage currents (see chapter 4).

Group 2

Group 2 comprises active implants. Once implanted, this kind of device is no longer accessible for maintenance purposes. For this reason safety must not depend on regular maintenance or corrective actions. Therefore, the process of designing and producing group 2 devices requires special quality assurance systems, including the implementation of a vigilance system (implanted pacemakers, implanted defibrillators, implanted drug delivery systems) that should make one aware of and able to react to design deficiencies.

Group 3

Group 3 contains all other active medical devices that have no increased risk but, because they are applied to patients, must provide enhanced safety compared with household devices (electrocardiogram recorders, ultrasound diagnostic devices, ergometers, etc.).

Group 4

Group 4 comprises all other nonactive devices that, depending on their use, might require regular checks, such as manual patient lifts or wheelchairs.

2 Law and Responsibility

2.1 Conscientiousness and Trust

Even if it is hard to believe—after looking at the newspapers or watching the TV news—a fundamental of social life is mutual trust. Every moment of life involves an element of trust: We rely on the safe construction and maintenance of the elevator we use; and on the right composition, hygienic production, and adequate storage of the food we eat. When driving, we rely on the correct behaviour of other drivers; in medicine in particular we must have trust in competent and efficient diagnosis, the right treatment, and, of course, the safe condition and application of medical devices.

Legislation has codified the principle that we can rely on the work of others. It obliges everybody to work with a reasonable amount of conscientiousness. A custodian who, after being advised otherwise, continues to use (electrical insulating) wax for the operation theatre's floor, which had initially and at high cost been made electrically conducting, fails in his duty; in the same way a surgeon fails when the patient is burned in high-frequency surgery because of a sloppily affixed neutral electrode.

**Trusting others obliges one's
own conscientiousness!**

Conscientiousness is more than working carefully: A service engineer who leaves his fingerprints, while adjusting the mirror in the beam pathway of therapy laser equipment, cannot justify the resulting damage by saying he did not know that high intensity laser radiation would cause burns at the site of fatty (burnable) fingerprints. Likewise, an electrician who still clamps soldered wires with screws, as he learned 20 years ago, violates his obligation to conscientiousness because safety standards no longer allow this practice.

Conscientiousness has two further consequences: First, it makes everyone responsible to keep their knowledge up to date. It is neither the duty of standardization organizations nor of the management of a company or hospital to say what people must learn. There is information provided, but the conclusions must be drawn by individuals themselves. Second, it is not possible to reject responsibility for one's work because of a lack of knowledge or experience. Everyone must only accept work for which they feel competent; otherwise they commit something called "acceptance negligence".

**Conscientiousness requires careful work,
full responsibility, and the continuous
and active updating of one's qualifications!**

Although there are many auto repair shops, a car driver must have basic technical knowledge of how to operate and maintain the car. Similarly, the presence of clinical engineers in hospitals does not mean that medical staff do not need to have a basic knowledge of medical technology.

In contrast to the situation in the USA, the requirements of professional qualification in Europe have far reaching consequences: In a recent situation in the USA a physician used high frequency surgery instead of a scalpel and caused severe burns. In the subsequent lawsuit the patient was awarded high damages. In this case, it was not the physician but the manufacturer of the high frequency surgical equipment who had to pay. The argument was that the instructions for use did not contain any warning that this method was not suitable for the performed type of surgery. In Europe the same case may have been treated as malpractice, because the physician who uses such surgical equipment is generally expected to have sufficient knowledge of its *intended use*.

Anybody who dries his wet pet in the microwave oven or who cuts his hedging with a lawn mower must (in Europe) assume responsibility. In case of harm, one is not only not allowed to bring claims, but can be charged with negligence, too.

It is the manufacturer who defines the intended use in the instructions for use: He states whether an infrared radiation device is intended for home use only or whether it might be used in a medical environment as well, and he indicates whether a device is intended to be used in an explosive atmosphere.

2.2 Technical Rules

Even if the names of national laws might be different in various countries, they all stipulate the obligation of the manufacturer to provide safe products. However, since total safety does not exist (see chapter 1), it is necessary to define the circumstances under which a product is considered to be sufficiently safe. This definition is made by safety standards. For economic reasons (and according to the European "New Approach" in 1985 and the following "Global Approach" in 1989) medical technology standards were different at various times. Today, within the 16 countries of the EU, there exists a hierarchical system of requirements that is composed of European directives with **mandatory** "essential requirements", as well as various technical standards that are voluntary **rules.** These standards are worked out by all 18 countries of the European Economic Space (European Union plus Norway and Switzerland) and are accepted by majority voting as European standards (EN) or European harmonizing documents (HD). All countries, even those that had been opposed to the standards originally, are obligated to adopt the standards and withdraw any national standards that conflict with the new documents.

2.2.1 Essential Requirements

Essential requirements are defined in the EU directives as general demands. Products placed on the market must be in conformity with them. Directives must be transformed into national laws to obtain mandatory legal status (e.g., directive 90/385/EEC on active medical implants or directive 93/42/EEC on medical devices). For medical devices these essential requirements comprise the following:

- **Safe design**

    — Choice of mechanically, chemically, and biologically suitable materials (e.g., according to the conditions of use, they must have stable shape, and be biocompatible, nontoxic, nonflammable, and nonaging)

- — Care for possible environmental conditions (e.g., temperature, humidity, liquid, electromagnetic interactions)

- — Prevention of excessive heating (e.g., by design, temperature control, cooling)

- — Care for hygienic aspects (e.g., by shaping, choice of materials, surface design, disinfectability)

- — Prevention of mechanical hazards (e.g., by ergonomic design, stability of the device, safety distances, breaking strength, and compression and crushing strength of the material used)

- — Protection against electrical shock (e.g., by sufficient insulation and separation of electrical circuits)

- — Protection against radiation hazards

- **Safe function**

  - — Warning for or prevention of dangerous outputs

  - — Measurement accuracy

  - — Reliability

- **Sufficient information**

  - — Instructions for use, labelling, and accompanying papers

- **Reliable production, packaging, transport, and storage**

2.2.2 Safety Standards

More detailed requirements are specified in the European standards. To not impede technical development, they are voluntary and have the status of technical rules: If they are fulfilled, the devices are considered to be in conformity with the (relevant) essential requirements. Manufacturers do not have to meet these rules word for word; the rules are flexible enough to allow for the development of alternative solutions with an equivalent degree of protection as well. What manufacturers are not allowed to do, however, is to provide a lower safety level than that defined in the standards. The development and change of standards are time-consuming procedures and, in general, are slower than technical progress. By this flexible approach the more rapid implementation of new technical developments should be encouraged.

For instance, up to 1988, IEC 601-1/1977 required that fuses not be soldered. This makes sense so as to allow the exchange of mains fuses rapidly and easily without further interference with the device. With time, manufacturers began to use cheap fuses to protect expensive electronic components by soldering them into electronic circuits like resistors. In this way such fuses did not prevent excessive heating or overload, but simply reduced repair costs. In countries such as Austria where IEC 601-1/1977 had a legal status, complaints were filed against these soldered fuses. The consequence was either to choose a time-consuming procedure to apply for an exception from the law for each type of equipment, or to remove such fuses—to the disadvantage of clients.

A survey of already-existing safety standards for medical electrical devices is given in Table 2.1. However, as the situation continuously changes, such surveys are not very current. Actual information, therefore, can be obtained from the responsible European or national institutions, which are summarized in Table 2.2.

In most cases the development of standards on international and national levels is done by two different organizations. At the global level these organizations are the International Electrotechnical Commission (IEC) for electrotechnical safety standards and the International Organization for Standardization (ISO) for general standards, both located in Geneva. They work out requirements that are not obligatory, but are intended to be guidelines for international harmonization. The related organizations at the European level are the Comité Européen de Normalisation Électrotechnique (CENELEC) and the Comité Européen de Normalisation (CEN), which are located in Brussels. They develop European standards that must be adopted by the member states. At the national level, mirror organizations like ÖVE and ON in Austria are in charge of standardization (Figure 2.1).

Active participation in this harmonization process is combined with a standstill obligation. As soon as standardization of a new work item is started at the European level, related work on individual national standards must be stopped. As a consequence, adoption of European standards is combined with the withdrawal of existing, conflicting national standards.

Device	International Standard	European standard
Medical electrical equipment—general requirements	IEC 601-1:1988 Ad. No. 1:1991	EN 60601-1:1990 + A1:1993 +A11:1993 +A12:1993 +A2:1995 +A13:1995
Medical electrical systems	IEC 601-1-1:1992 Ad. No.1:1995	EN 60601-1-1:1993 +A1:1996
Electromagnetic compatibility	IEC 601-1-2:1993	EN 60601-1-2:1993
Radiation protection in diagnostic X-ray equipment	IEC 601-1-3:1994	EN 60601-1-3:1994
Programmable electronic systems	IEC 601-1-4	EN 60601-1-4
Medical electron accelerators	IEC 601-2-1:1981 Ad. No. 1:1984 Ad. No. 2:1990	

Table 2.1. Survey on Safety Standards for Medical Electrical Equipment (as of March 1996).

Table 2.1 continued.

Device	International Standard	European standard
High frequency surgical equipment	IEC 601-2-2:1991	EN 60601-2-2:1993
Shortwave therapy equipment	IEC 601-2-3:1991	EN 60601-2-3:1993
Cardiac defibrillators/monitors	IEC 601-2-4:1983	HD 395.2.4 S1:1988
Ultrasonic therapy equipment	IEC 601-2-5:1984	HD 395.2.5 S1:1986
Microwave therapy equipment	IEC 601-2-6:1984	HD 395.2.6 S1:1986
Diagnostic X-ray generators	IEC 601-2-7:1987	HD 395.2.7 S1:1989
Therapeutic X-ray generators	IEC 601-2-8:1987	HD 395.2.8 S1:1988
Dosimeters used in radiotherapy	IEC 601-2-9:1987	HD 395.2.9 S1:1988
Nerve and muscle stimulators	IEC 601-2-10:1987	HD 395.2.10 S1:1989
Gamma beam therapy equipment	IEC 601-2-11:1987 Ad. No. 1:1988	HD 395.2.11 S2:1990

Table 2.1 continued on next page.

Table 2.1 continued.

Device	International Standard	European standard
Lung ventilators for medical use	IEC 601-2-12:1988	EN 794:1996
Anaesthetic machines	IEC 601-2-13:1989	HD 395.2.13 S1:1989 EN 740:1995
Electroconvulsive therapy equipment	IEC 601-2-14:1989	HD 395.2.14 S1:1989
Capacitor discharge X-ray generators	IEC 601-2-15:1988	HD 395.2.15 S1:1989
Haemodialysis equipment	IEC 601-2-16:1989	HD 395.2.16 S1:1989
Gamma-ray afterloading equipment	IEC 601-2-17:1989	HD 395.2.17 S1:1992
Endoscopic equipment	IEC 601-2-18:1990	EN 60601-2-18:1995
Baby incubators	IEC 601-2-19:1990	EN 60601-2-19:1995
Transport incubators	IEC 601-2-20:1990	EN 60601-2-20:1995
Infant radiation warmers	IEC 601-2-21:1994	EN 60601-2-21:1994

Table 2.1 continued on next page.

Table 2.1 continued.

Device	International Standard	European standard
Diagnostic and therapeutic laser equipment	IEC 601-2-22:1992	EN 60601-2-22:1992
Transcutaneous partial pressure monitoring equipment	IEC 601-2-23:1993	
Infusion pumps	Draft IEC 601-2-24:1994	prHD 395-2-24:1994
Electrocardiographs	IEC 601-2-25:1993	EN 60601-2-25:1995
Electroencephalographs	IEC 601-2-26:1994	EN 60601-2-26:1994
ECG monitoring equipment	IEC 601-2-27:1994	EN 60601-2-27:1994
X-ray source assemblies and X-ray tube assemblies	IEC 601-2-28:1993	EN 60601-2-28:1993
Radiotherapy simulators	IEC 601-2-29:1993	EN 60601-2-29:1995
Cyclic indirect blood-pressure monitoring equipment	IEC 601-2-30:1995	EN 60601-2-30:1995
External cardiac pacemakers	IEC 601-2-31:1994	EN 60601-2-31:1995

Table 2.1 continued on next page.

Table 2.1 continued.

Device	International Standard	European standard
X-ray equipment	IEC 601-2-32:1994	EN 60601-2-32:1995
Magnetic resonance imaging equipment	IEC 601-2-33:1995	EN 60601-2-33:1995
Direct blood-pressure monitoring equipment	IEC 601-2-34:1994	EN 60601-2-34:1995
Heating blankets	IEC 601-2-35:1994	
Extracorporally induced lithotripsy	IEC 601-2-36:1995	
Ultrasonic diagnostic and monitoring equipment	(Draft IEC 601-2-37)	
Hospital beds	IEC 601-2-38:1995	prEN 50079
Peritoneal dialysis equipment	IEC 601-2-39:1995	EN 50072:1992
Electromyographs and evoked response systems	(Draft IEC 601-2-40)	
Operating table luminaire	Draft IEC 601-2-41:1995	

Table 2.1 continued on next page.

Table 2.1 continued.

Device	International Standard	European standard
Automatic external defibrillators	(Draft IEC 601-2-42)	
X-ray equipment for interventional radiography	(Draft IEC 601-2-43)	
X-ray computer tomography	(Draft IEC 601-2-44)	
X-ray mammography equipment	(Draft IEC 601-2-45)	
Operating tables	Draft IEC 601-2-46:1995	prEN 50115:1993
Electrically powered suction equipment	Draft ISO 10079/1994	
Implantable cardiac pacemakers	ISO 5841-1:1989	EN 50061:1988 + A1: 1991
Electrical equipment with electric patient circuits (home use equipment)	(Draft IEC 1814)	
Electrical equipment for measurement, control and laboratory use—general requirements	IEC 1010-1:1990 + Ad. No. 1:1992	EN 61010-1:1993

Country	Abbreviation	Organization	Address
	IEC	International Electrotechnical Commission	3, Rue de Varembè, P.O.Box 131 CH - 1211 Genf
	ISO	International Organization for Standardization	3, Rue de Varembè, P.O.Box 131 CH - 1211 Genf
	CENELEC	Comité Européen de Normalisation Électrotechnique	2, Rue Brederode BTE 5 B - 1000 Brüssel
	CEN	Comité Européen de Normalisation	2, Rue Brederode BTE 5 B - 1000 Brüssel
A	ÖKE	Österreichisches Kommittee für Elektrotechnik	Eschenbachgasse 9 A - 1010 Wien
	ON	Österreichisches Normungsinstitut	Heinestraße 38 A - 1021 Wien
B	CEB	Le Comité Electrotechnique Belge	3 Galèrie Ravenstein B - 1000 Brüssel

Table 2.2. National and International Institutions Responsible for Standardization

Table 2.2 continued.

Country	Abbreviation	Organization	Address
	IBN	Institut Belge de Normalisation	29 Avenue de la Barbauconne B - 1040 Brüssel
CH	CES	Comité Electrotechnique Suisse	Seefeldstraße 301 CH - 8034 Zürich
	SNV	Schweizerische Normen - Vereinigung	Luppmenstraße 1 CH - 8320 Fehraltorf
D	DKE	Deutsche Elektrotechnische Kommission	Stresemannallee 15 D - 60596 Frankfurt 70
	DIN	Deutsches Institut für Normen e.V.	Burggrafenstraße 6, Postfach 1107 D - 1000 Berlin 30
DK	DEMKO	Danmarks Elektriske Materiel - Kontrol	Lyskaer 8 DK - 2730 Herlev

Table 2.2 continued on next page.

Table 2.2 continued.

Country	Abbreviation	Organization	Address
	DS	Dansk Standardiseringsrad	Baunegaardvej 73 DK - 2900 Hellerup
E	AEE	Associaciòn Electrotécnica y Electrònica Espaniole	Avenida del' Brasil 7 E - 28020 Madrid
	AENOR	Associaciòn Espaniola de Normalizacion y Certificacion	Fernandez de la Hoz 52 E - 28010 Madrid
F	UTE	Union Technique de l'Electricité	UTE Cedex 64 F - 92052 Paris La Defense
	AFNOR	Association Francaise de Normalisation	Tour Europe - Cedex F - 92049 Paris La Defense
GB	BEC	British Electrotechnical Committee	c/o BSI
	BSI	British Standards Institute	2 Park Street GB - London WIA 2 BS

Table 2.2 continued on next page.

Table 2.2 continued.

Country	Abbreviation	Organization	Address
GR	ELOT	Ellinicos Organismos Typopoiiseos	313 Archanon GR - 11145 Athen
I	CEI	Comitato Elettrotecnico Italiano	Via Monza 259 I - 20126 Mailand
	UNI	Ente Nationale Italiano di Unificazione	Piazza Armando Diaz 2 I - 20123 Mailand
IRL	ETCI	Electrotechnical Council of Ireland	Parnell Av., Harold's Cross IRL - Dublin 12
	NSAI	National Standards Authority of Ireland	Ballymun road IRL - Dublin 9
IS	STRI	Technological Institute of Iceland	c/o STRI
		Standardization Council of Iceland	Keldnaholt IS - 112 Reykjavik

Table 2.2 continued on next page.

Table 2.2 continued.

Country	Abbreviation	Organization	Address
L	SEE	Service de l'Energie de l'Etat	Avenue de la Porte Neuve 34 L - 2132 Luxemburg
	ITM	Inspection des Travail et des Mines	26 rue Zithe, BP. 27 L - 2010 Luxemburg
N	NEK	Norsk Elektrotechnisk Komite	Harbitzalleen 2A, Skoyen PB 280 N - 0212 Oslo 2
	NSF	Norges Standardiseringsforbund	Postboks 7020 Hormansbyer N - 0306 Oslo 3
NL	NEC	Nederlands Elektrotechnisch Comité	Kalfjeslaan 2, Postbus 5059 NL - 2600 GB Delft
	NNI	Nederlands Normalisatie Institut	Kalfjeslaan 2, Postbus 5059 NL - 2600 GB Delft

Table 2.2 continued on next page.

Table 2.2 continued.

Country	Abbreviation	Organization	Address
P	IPQ	Instituto Portugès da Qualidade	Rue Jose Estevao 83A P - 1199 Lissabon Codex
S	SEK	Svenska Elektriska Kommissionen	Kistagangen 19, Box 1284 S - 16428 Kista Stockholm
	SIS	Standeriseringskommissionen i Sverige	Box 3295 - Tenergatan 11 S - 10366 Stockholm
SF	SESKO	Finish Electrotechnical Standards Association	P.O. Box 134 SF - 00211 Helsinki 21
	SFS	Suomen Standardissimisliitto t. y.	P.O. Box 205, Bulevardi 5A7 SF - 00121 Helsinki

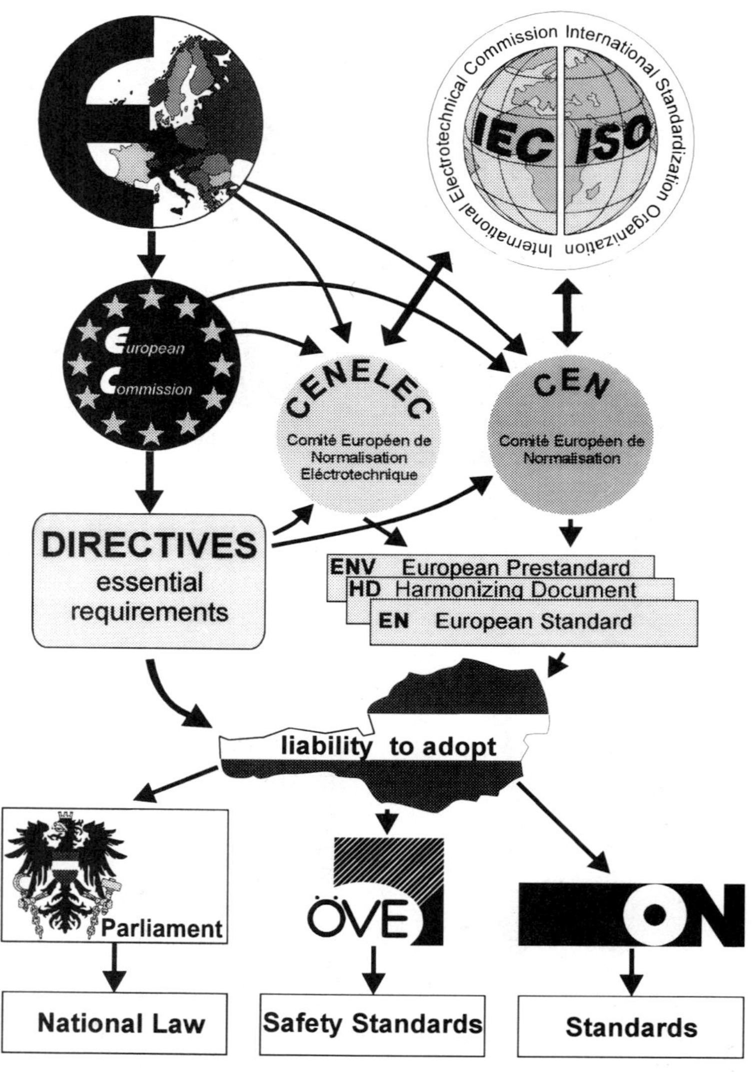

Figure 2.1. Organization of standardization at global (IEC, ISO), European (CENELEC, CEN), and national (ÖVE, ON) levels.

The result of this procedure is that standards for medical electrical devices are already harmonized throughout Europe. Therefore, a manufacturer can no longer refuse to bring his device into line with safety requirements by using the argument that, for economic reasons, it could not respond to the extra wishes of every individual (small) country.

Safety requirements for medical electrical devices are already harmonized!

In fact, for manufacturers the situation is even more favorable: European standards for medical devices in general fully comply with the IEC standards (Table 2.1) and, therefore, harmonization extends beyond European boundaries. Since IEC standards are voluntary only, it must be added that even countries like the USA, who once voted in favor of IEC standards, still may have their own conflicting (e.g., FDA) regulations.

2.3 Why Testing?

We can trust that manufacturers will produce devices that not only have the claimed performance but also comply with the safety standards. Experience, however, shows that confidence is oftentimes unjustified. In fact, most of the tested devices do not pass safety tests without modifications, even if they are new. Therefore, particularly in medical device technology, the proof of safety by a test certificate of an accredited test house is strongly recommended.

Most (untested) devices do not comply with safety standards!

To make a further step toward a free market and to improve competitiveness, the European Medical Device Directive 93/42/EEC allows all devices to be put on the market if they are in conformity with the essential requirements. This must be indicated by the CE mark (Figure 2.2). It must be stressed that this label does not constitute proof of either quality or safety. According to its intent, it is addressed to the national authorities, not to the customer. It merely indicates that marketing a device must not be impeded. As a consequence, the requirements for its attachment may not include testing by independent test houses.

To define the conformity assessment requirements, the entire field of medical devices, from adhesive strips to heart-lung machines, from condoms to computer tomography, is classified according to 18 rules in 4 product groups with respect to the invasiveness of products as well as the potential hazards of their methods of application and the duration of their use (Figure 2.3).

1.   **Group I** comprises devices that are characterized by low invasiveness—no or uncritical

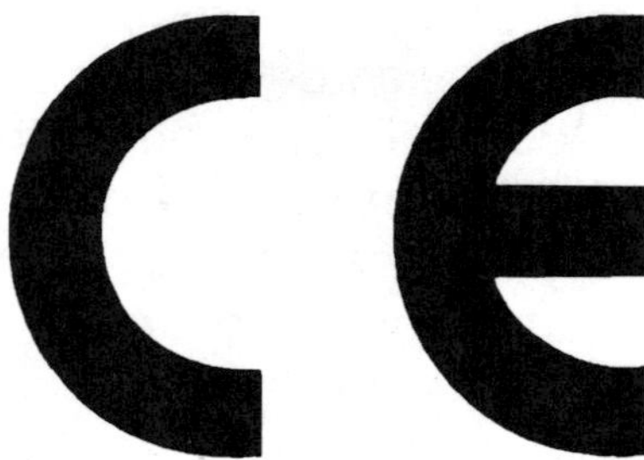

Figure 2.2. European conformity mark.

Figure 2.3. Survey of the conformity classification procedures for medical devices.

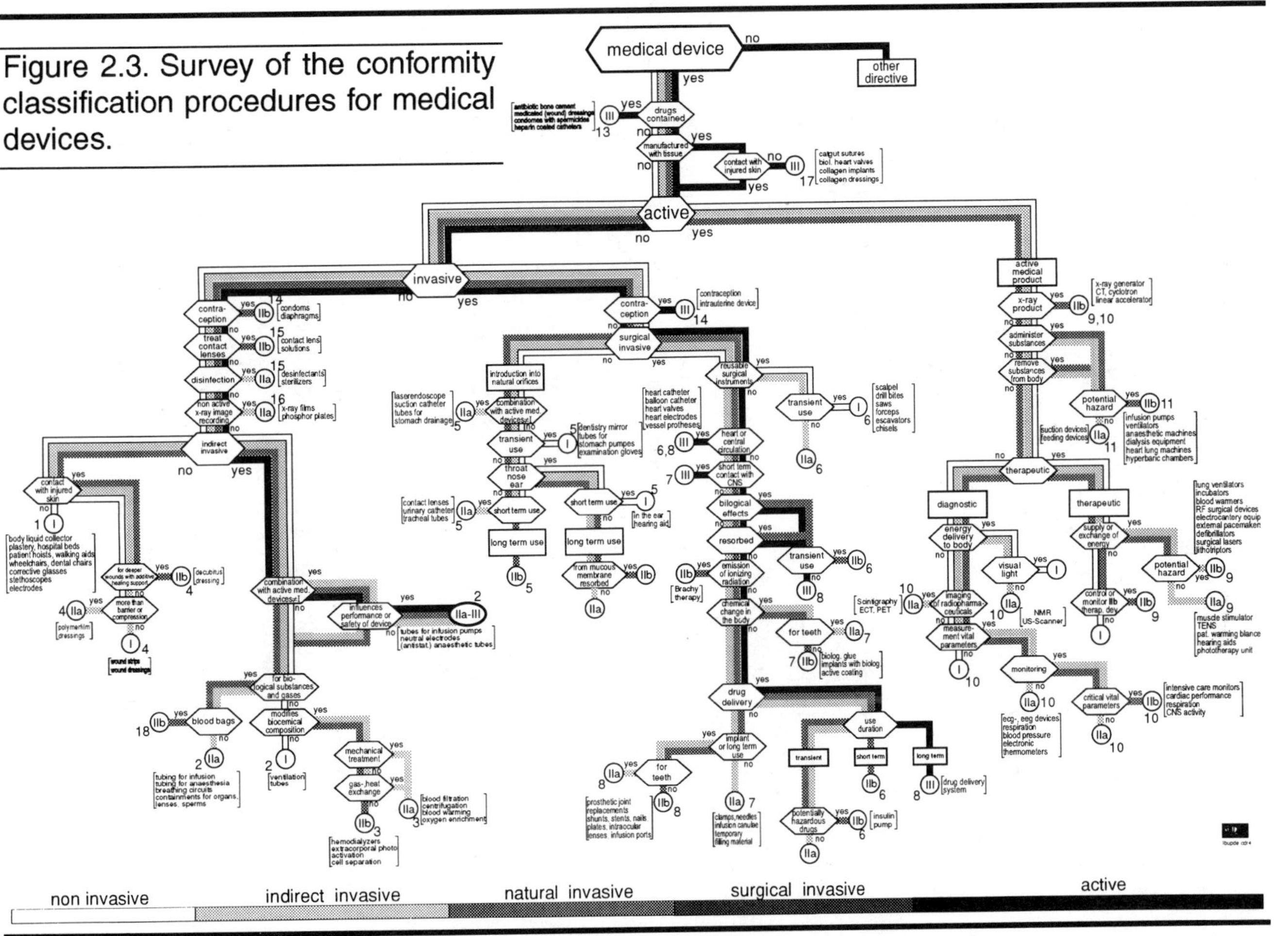

contact with the skin, no potential methodological hazards—and are intended for transient use (less than one hour) only (e.g., infrared thermography equipment, bicycle ergometers, electrocardiogram recorders, and thermometers).

2. **Group IIa** consists of devices that are characterized by medium invasiveness, potential methodological hazards, short-term use (less than one month), and application at natural or surgical orifices (e.g., ultrasound imagers, suction devices, inhalators, blood pumps, nerve and muscle stimulators, and diathermy equipment).

3. **Group IIb** includes devices with increased potential methodological hazards, and that have systemic effects or are intended for long-term use (more than one month) (e.g., X-ray devices, laser equipment, lithotriptors, defibrillators, incubators, heart-lung machines, and heart and blood circulation monitors). This group also includes devices for noninvasive contraception.

4. **Group III** comprises devices for direct application in the open heart or the central nervous system, with possibly enhanced methodological hazards, or for long-term drug delivery (e.g., active implants, such as pacemakers, insulin pumps, and heart valves). This group also includes products for natural invasive contraception.

2.3.1 Conformity Assessment

In principle, every medical device must be tested to determine if it meets the essential requirements. The manufacturer must include these test results with the product file of a device. In regard to the involvement of external bodies, however, conformity assessment requirements are quite different. In the largest group (group I) the manufacturer can perform his own testing and mark his device without the need for further external testing. Group IIa devices additionally require some quality assurance of the production process that must be certified by a notified body. Only group IIb and III devices must be tested by a notified body, either directly by EC type testing or indirectly by full quality assurance assessment according to EN 46001 (Figure 2.4).

The disadvantage of the CE marking is that it is not intended to indicate proven safety. The overwhelming numbers of medical devices, however, fall into group I or IIa and, therefore, are declared to be in conformity with the essential requirements by the manufacturer itself without any independent safety test. However, if the device is poorly designed, the assessment of the production quality system cannot improve its safety. It only assures the reliable multiplication of (even unsafe) devices. Only if a device bears a safety mark (or is group IIb) is there evidence that it is safe (Figure 2.5).

CE marking does not indicate proof of safety!

The recommendation to ask for a test certificate is not given without reason. The lifetime average of medical

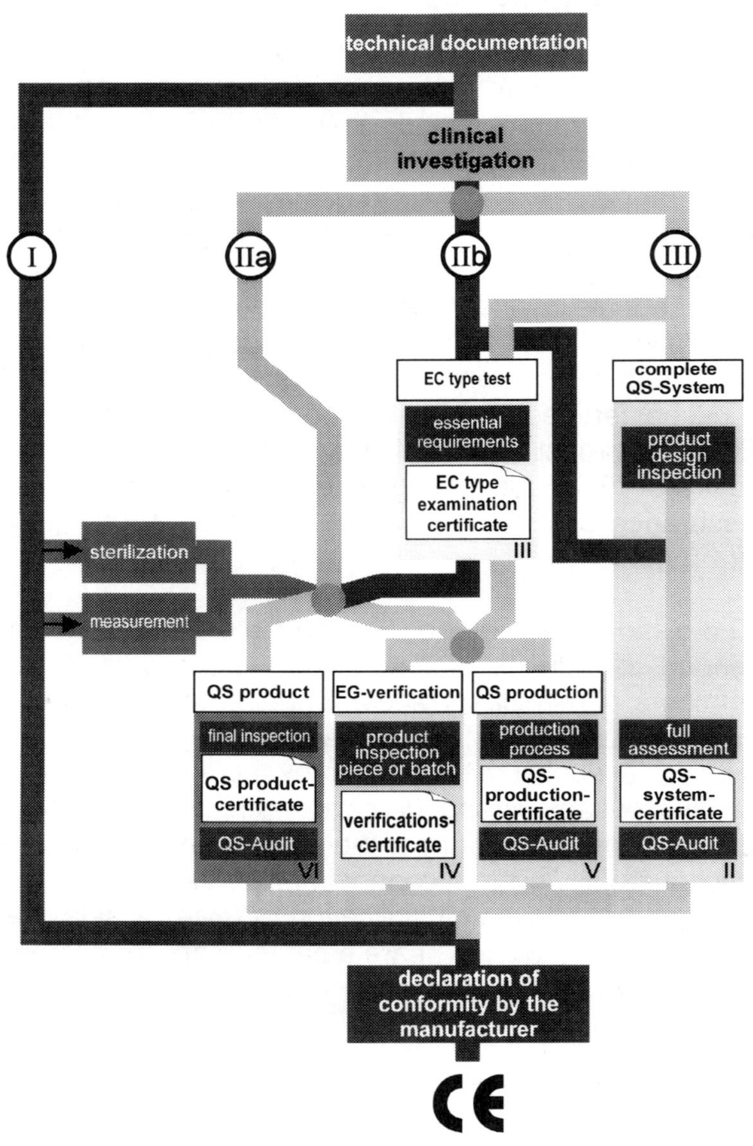

Figure 2.4. Conformity assessment requirements.

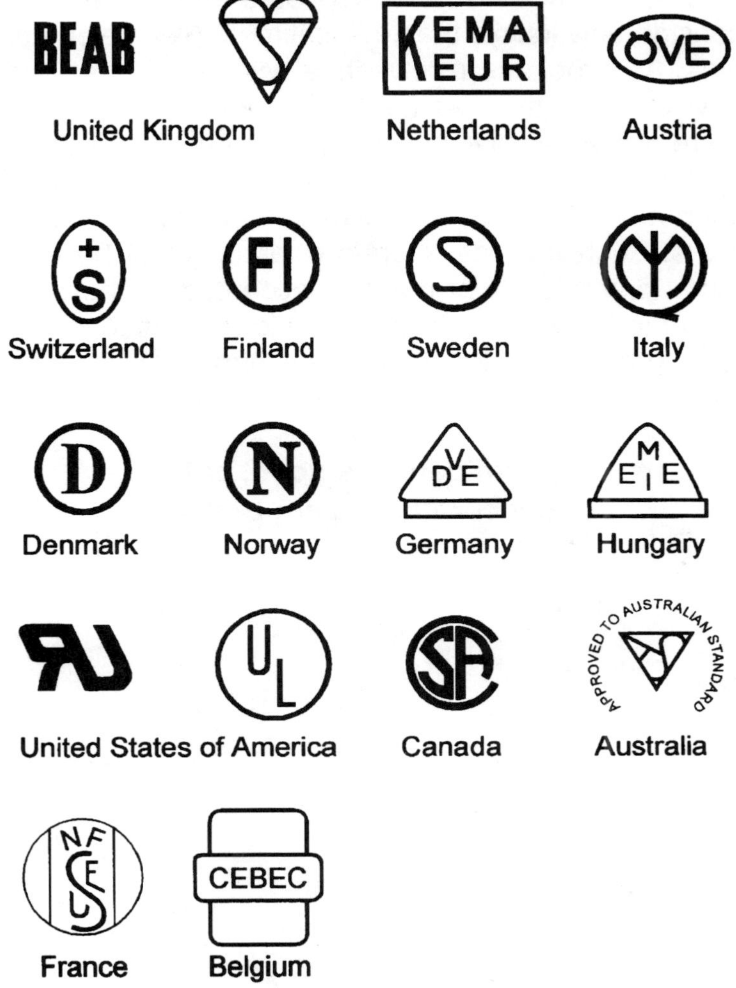

Figure 2.5. National safety marks.

electrical devices is 10 to 15 years and, therefore, is considerably longer than the lifetimes of some companies. As problems rarely arise with poorly designed devices when they are new, the probability is high that there will be no one to contact when the need arises. Furthermore, most design-related safety problems cannot be solved without compromises and additional costs. Such devices, therefore, either must be eliminated prematurely or must be accepted as they were from the beginning: as problematic devices that make life more difficult for all involved parties. This, therefore, leads to the following recommendation:

**Confidence is good, but
test certificates are better!**

3 The Basic Principles of Electrotechnology

It is not possible to understand the safety aspects of electromedical devices without at least a basic knowledge of the main principles of electricity. There is a surprising analogy between electric circuits and water flow that makes understanding electricity easier. By examining this analogy, the concepts of electric charge, voltage, current, and resistance are explained in this chapter, and beginning insights into safety problems are presented.

3.1 Charge and Voltage

Electricity has much in common with truth: Everybody talks about it, but nobody really knows it. Today, we know that electricity is a fundamental phenomenon of nature inherent in the very existence of matter. Every material is composed of atoms consisting of positively charged nuclei surrounded by a cloud of negatively charged electrons. We know the effects of electricity and succeed in making its forces usable as far as possible, but the question of what its final nature is remains open. We know that electrical phenomena are caused by something we call **"charges"**, and that there are two different kinds of charges that since the 18th century (and without any intention of making value judgments) have been called "positive" and "negative". We also know that different materials contain different amounts of charges. This is the reason we may experience annoying discharges when we get out of a plastic chair: At the area where different materials are in contact, electric charges are exchanged until an equilibrium is reached. When we stand up, because of the low conductivity, the charges on the plastic chair do not have enough time to move back and, therefore, cause a surplus that may be discharged by the emission of a spark.

In ancient Greece there were, of course, no plastic chairs, but people already knew that amber could be brought into a different status by rubbing it with some wool. This explains the origin of the term *electricity:* It is derived from the Greek word for amber, "elektron".

Electrical charging by rubbing is common in everyday life. It can also become a severe safety problem. Depending on their clothing, people can charge themselves by moving their arms or legs. In this way they can accumulate electric charges to an extent that in operation theatres is far more than sufficient to cause explosions through the ignition of flammable mixtures, like anaesthetic gases. This is the reason several antistatic measures are necessary.

Although we do not know the final nature of electric charges, we have very detailed knowledge of how they behave: They are quite similar to other things in life, where opposites attract and identical entities repel each other. This can be formulated as the following important principle:

Opposite electric charges attract each other; identical electric charges repel each other!

The principle of attraction and repulsion holds in nearly all electrotechnical applications. But once two different charges are combined, something amazing happens. In a surprising magic trick of nature, they suddenly disappear from the (electric) scene as if they had never been there before: A pair of opposite electrical charges behaves as if it were electrically neutral.

However, separating a pair of opposite electric charges is laborious: It requires work (which must be done, for example, in power plants) and is not finished with mere separation, because an electric **voltage** exists between the separated charges, which can be described as the tendency of recombination. Voltage increases with the number of separated charges.

Especially in regard to the terms *electric voltage* and *electric current,* there is still a Tower of Babylon–like confusion. It is important to emphasize that the existence of an electric voltage does not necessarily produce an electric current, but it is a requirement of such a possible effect that also depends on other factors.

**Electric voltage is just a condition and
not an effect as such!**

Probably you are not aware that while taking a shower, you have much in common with persons exposed to an electric shock. But, in fact, the fundamental principles of water flow and electric current flow are quite similar. Electrical effects, therefore, can be illustrated by taking advantage of this analogy and by considering the following terms as similar to each other (Figure 3.1):

electric charge ↔ water drop

electric voltage ↔ water pressure (height difference)

electric potential ↔ height

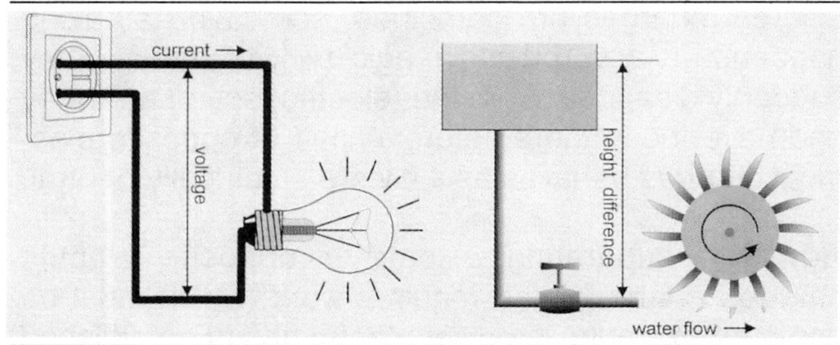

Figure 3.1. Analogy of electrical and hydraulic principles.

electric current ↔ water flow

electric resistance ↔ flow resistance

electric lead ↔ water tube

A battery or a mains socket outlet has poles where charges are accumulated. This can be compared with a dam behind which water is collected. The thickness of the dam is dependent on the height difference from the water level to the ground. Likewise, the thickness of the required electrical insulation is determined by the electric voltage. Beware, however, if the dam breaks and the water floods the valley. It is similar with electric voltage: An insulation failure would cause an instantaneous reunion of the "stored" electric charges. The consequences of the resulting short circuit depend on the number of charges involved. The accessible amount of electric charges, however, is nearly infinite at mains socket outlets compared with batteries, so mains circuits ultimately require means (fuses) that act as charge limiters.

Whether there will be a disastrous flood or whether the water will be used under control to run a generator depends not only on the height difference but also on other circumstances. Similarly, the electric voltage determines the potential for hazard; whether there will be damage or a useful application is dependent on further conditions.

The electric voltage determines the potential for a hazard!

For safety considerations this means that risk can be reduced if the voltage is decreased. This is the reason, especially in America, mains voltage has been set at half the value of that in Europe (Figure 3.2). For the same reason it is necessary by different means to take strict care to avoid the appearance of unintended voltages in operation theatres (see chapter 4).

If you are watering flowers with a garden hose, you use the same laws that are valid for electric circuits:

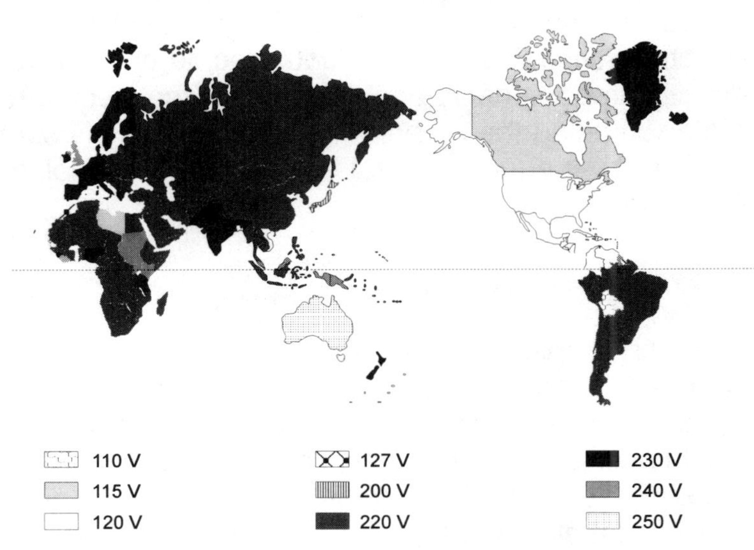

Figure 3.2. Worldwide mains voltage amplitudes.

The hose is under constant pressure. Whether flowers are gently watered or damaged by an intense water jet is dependent on the amount of water and its flow velocity. Likewise, the effect of electricity on people is dependent on the amount of electric charges and their velocity. These factors are summarized by the term *electric current.*

**The electric current determines
the (biological) effect!**

The prevention of damage, therefore, requires that currents be limited by some safety means, such as automatic cutouts or fuses in feeder boxes.

3.2 Ohm's Law and Safety

At constant pressure, water jet strength is dependent on how far you have opened the hose and thus reduced the flow resistance. In a similar way the cause (electric voltage) and the effect (electric current) are directly proportional to each other, with the electric **resistance** being the proportionality factor. This is summarized by the fundamental law of electrotechnology, Ohm's law:

$$\textbf{current} = \frac{\textbf{voltage}}{\textbf{resistance}}$$

Although simple, this relation has considerable consequences: It means that electric voltages would require an enormously high (infinite!) resistance to prevent electric currents from flowing. However, insulating material with such an ideal resistance does not exist. It follows that electric (leakage) currents cannot, in principle, be avoided and can be found in everyday life.

Electric (leakage) currents are omnipresent!

The second consequence of Ohm's law is that the hazard increases if the resistance is reduced. If the electric resistance of our insulating dry skin is reduced because it becomes wet while bathing or cooking, then the protection against electric shock is reduced. The most dangerous situation can be found in operation theatres, where the body of the patient is opened and his skin can no longer protect him (see Figure 4.8). In contrast, electrical safety is increased if the insulating property of the skin is enhanced (e.g., by fatty creams, or by wearing rubber gloves, as when doing household work or surgery).

Ohm's law can also be written in a different way:

voltage = current × resistance

At first glance it might not be obvious that important conclusions follow from this simple relation as well. It must be taken into account that just as there are no ideal insulators, in daily life there are no ideal conductors either. Therefore, it follows that as soon as currents flow, they cause electric voltages and develop new hazard potentials. We have already stated that electric currents are omnipresent. Now we must accept that this applies to electric voltages as well. In some cases they might reach such high levels that further actions are needed.

Electric voltages are omnipresent!

In spite of intact protection, people, even within their homes, might be killed by a lightning strike. This can be explained by Ohm's law: Lightning currents can reach amplitudes as high as 500,000 A. If a high current flows across a low ground resistance (0.1 Ω) of an electrical installation, according to Ohm's law, this can cause voltages as high as 50,000 V. Therefore, high voltages can appear between protectively earthed electrical devices and other grounded parts (such as water pipes and heating bodies) that the lightning current did not flow through and, therefore, remained at ground potential. To avoid such hazardous situations, it is mandatory to connect the grounded parts of an electrical installation together with other grounded parts in a house (potential equalization).

Comparatively low voltages can cause hazards in operation theatres (see chapter 4). However, potential differences between the various devices are unavoidable. They may be caused by different lengths of the supply cord, different currents, or different connection sites within the electrical circuit. This makes special precautions (special potential equalization) necessary.

There is one apparent contradiction to be resolved: If you are carrying a car battery and touch the positive pole, no current is flowing across your body. However, as soon as the battery is installed in a car and you touch the same positive pole, a current will flow! This observation is of considerable importance. Currents can flow only if the electrical circuit is closed. This means that the charges of one pole must have the possibility to recombine with the separated charges of the counterpole!

Electric currents can flow in closed circuits only!

While you were carrying the battery, the second pole was without contact and, therefore, the circuit across your body was open. The fact that the current did flow after installation, although you again only touched the positive pole, is not in contradiction with the above statement: The negative pole of the car battery is connected with the coachwork and thereby with ground potential. Because persons are considered to be grounded in safety discussions, current is flowing from the positive pole across your body to the ground and from this to the grounded negative pole—there now is a closed loop.

For safety considerations persons are considered to be grounded!

The apparently trivial condition that circuits must be closed to allow electric currents to flow has two important consequences. It can mean an opportunity as well as a danger.

The *opportunity* is an important safety strategy: If both poles of an electric source are insulated from the earth, a person (who is considered to be earthed) is still protected if he accidentally comes into contact with one of the poles, because the circuit still remains open. This is not a theoretical subtlety. In fact, this method has been chosen to improve safety in operation theatres: By using a separating transformer, both poles of the electric source are insulated from the ground. Thus, two things are accomplished: Besides the improvement of protection against electrical shock, an unintended contact with the earth (e.g., due to an insulation failure) does not cause a short circuit. Therefore, activating a circuit breaker and interrupting the power supply at all mains socket outlets of the same circuit can be avoided. Insulated power supply allows electrical devices to continue working, even under first failure conditions, which is of special importance if life-saving electromedical devices are being used.

The *dangerous* consequence of the closed circuit condition stems from the fact that electric currents follow all possible circuit paths to reach the counterpole—not only the intended one. Ohm's law demonstrates that it is not possible to prevent current from flowing even across dedicated electric insulation. This means there are many possible circuit paths that must be taken into account. As in rush hour when traffic uses even small side streets to move forward, electric currents use any route to flow back and, of course, are also flowing across the patient, where the electric resistance is the lowest.

Electric currents follow all possible circuit paths to the counterpole!

This fact is especially important for patients who simultaneously are connected to several electromedical devices, such as an electrocardiogram monitor, a blood gas monitor, a suction device, a high frequency surgery device, and an anaesthetic machine. In the case of grounded patient circuits (Figure 3.3), currents not only flow as intended from one electrode to the other, but also use various pathways to other applied parts, to earthed housings of devices, to accidentally touched grounded metallic holders, to the operating table, and so forth. This complicated pattern of current pathways significantly increases the risk for fibrillation and unintended burns (see chapter 4). This is the reason electric circuits intended to include the patient (as in nerve and muscle stimulators, high frequency surgical devices, etc.) must be insulated from the earth as a precaution.

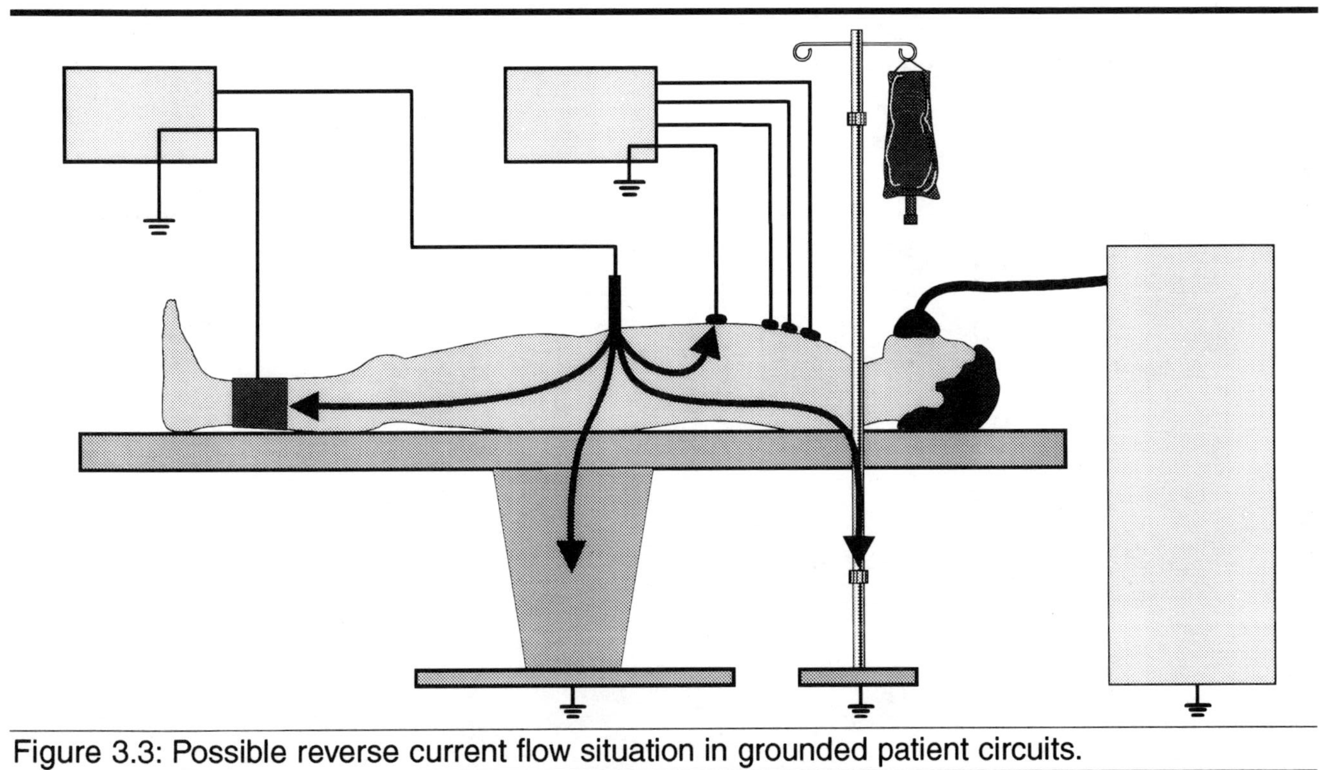

Figure 3.3: Possible reverse current flow situation in grounded patient circuits.

4 Electric Current Effects

Very few people have not experienced an electrical shock due to contact with dangerous voltages. There are two reasons electrical accidents are comparatively rare: (1) Our *reaction,* which generally allows us to end the contact with live parts (this already demonstrates that hazards are considerably dependent on contact duration!) and (2) electrical *protective means,* which protect us from danger.

In this chapter electric current is shown to be responsible for the biological consequences of an accident. Further, the chapter describes the considerations and assumptions that allow the derivation of safe voltage limits based on electric current bioeffects. This will help explain why voltages in operation theatres are considered dangerous even though they are less than one-thousandth of the voltages children may be exposed to when playing with electric toy trains.

4.1 Cellular Excitation

More than 200 years ago, in 1791, Galilei described a ghostly experiment: He noted that by electric discharges a dead frog's thigh could apparently be brought to life and to make convulsive movements. Today, we know that electrical phenomena for our bodies are nothing new. We know that physiological processes are essentially based on electrical effects, which are strong enough to be observed at the body's surface. This is useful in medicine, since it allows us to monitor the action of internal organs by measuring their electric signals with surface electrodes (e.g., electrocardiograms of the heart, electroencephalograms of the brain, electromyograms of the muscles, and electroretinograms of the eye). One reason is that our body is electrically conducting. This means that it contains many free, movable, electric charges of both polarities that permit a change of the electric surface potential at the skin according to internal electric processes. Another reason can be found in the electrical properties of our cell membranes: In principle, cell membranes are good electrical insulators. However, they exhibit different behaviour in respect to different kinds of electrically charged particles, which they allow to penetrate in different ways. This results in an unbalanced distribution of electric charges; under steady state conditions there is a surplus of negative charges inside the cell and a surplus of positive charges outside. Thus, each cell effectively becomes an electric battery with a voltage of about 90 mV.

Nerve and muscle cells are characterized by the fact that this electrical steady state condition can change dramatically. If negative electric charges are brought into the extracellular space, they compensate for the surplus of positive charges and reduce the membrane voltage. At the beginning, this has no special effect, but if a certain amount of voltage reduction (the excitation threshold) is exceeded (which occurs at a change of about 20 percent), the insulating properties of the membrane break down dramatically, allowing a sudden equalization of intra- and extracellular charges. This results in a sudden peak of the membrane voltage, called an "action potential". Afterward, the steady state is slowly restored by active transport processes that remove the surplus of intracellular charged particles. This excitation process obeys the "all or nothing" rule, which means that once the excitation threshold is exceeded, excitation always is maximum and is not influenced by the strength of the stimulus.

The electrical impulse of the excitation can also be transmitted. In nerve cells it propagates along the nerve fiber; in heart cells excitation is passed forward from cell to cell, as in a game of dominoes.

To excite a cell, the stimulus (i.e., the electric current), must fulfill three conditions: (1) It must be **strong enough** to exceed the excitation threshold; (2) its duration must be **long enough** to allow cellular processes to be activated before it diminishes again; (3) it must **change rapidly enough** to prevent cellular states from adapting without excitation.

**Excitatory stimuli need strength,
duration, and change!**

With sinusoidal currents, the positive (excitatory) half wave is followed by the negative (inhibiting) half wave and vice versa. The stimulus duration, therefore, is directly dependent on the frequency of the electric current; thus, the excitability of electric currents is frequency dependent. It decreases with increasing frequency until even large currents are no longer able to excite cells. Above 100 kHz biologic effects are based on heating only. This is why high frequencies of about 400 kHz are used in electrosurgery. They allow utilization of thermal effects to cut and coagulate tissue, without causing convulsive movements of the patient.

At the low frequency end of the spectrum, sensitivity to excitation decreases again, this time because of the slow change of the stimulus. Indeed, direct current can influence excitability, but cannot excite cells unless during on or off switching. This is why direct currents are less hazardous than sinusoidal currents.

Unfortunately, our mains frequency belongs to the biologically most effective frequency range, in which cells are most sensitive to excitation. The biological effects of electric currents also depend considerably on the affected site, as well as on the thickness and composition of the skin. In addition, sensitivity to electric currents is quite different from person to person. The range of mains current perception thresholds for a current pathway from hand to hand amounts to a factor of 10; if currents are applied to the lower arm only, the range is increased to a factor of 100 (Figure 4.1).

4.2 Heart Fibrillation

Saying that someone's "heart can break", that someone has a "heart of stone", that the "heart can sink", that we "wear our heart on our sleeve" or even "lose our heart" reminds us that for a long time the heart was believed to bear someone's feelings or even the soul. Therefore, it was not surprising that heart transplants, which today are almost routine, initially had to overcome great emotional and ethical concerns, and for some patients even led to an identity crisis.

Today, the situation is cleared up: We see the heart in a more unemotional way, namely, just as a pump, although a special one, on whose reliable function our life depends. In principle, our heart is considered to be

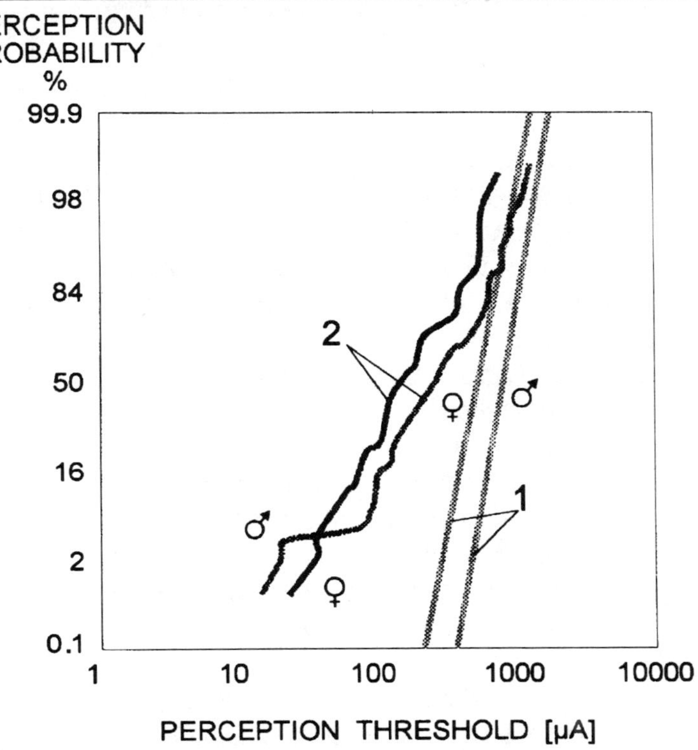

Figure 4.1. Perception threshold for mains frequency currency flowing from hand to hand (Dalziel 1961) and if applied to the lower arm only (Leitgeb 1995).

a mechanical organ that must fulfill a simple task. To be able to perform its pumping action with the necessary reliability, our heart makes use of four special properties:

1.   *Autonomous excitation:* This is demonstrated by Cortez' conquest of Mexico in the 16th century: The reports describe sacrifices in which the sacrificer offers to his god the

victim's heart, which is continuing its action although it has already been removed from the body. The fact that the heart continues pumping, although disconnected from the brain, demonstrates the heart's first property—the ability to undergo **autonomous excitation.** This means that the heart is provided with its own excitation center—cells that are able to self-excite in a certain rhythm.

2.   *Excitation distributes:* In contrast to skeletal muscle cells, heart muscle cells are able to **pass on their excitation** to neighbouring cells. Essentially, after being initiated by the excitation center, stimulation is distributed over the whole heart in a chain reaction, as when a row of dominoes falls after the first one is knocked down.

3.   *Excitation propagation system:* Pumping requires more than just the excitation of muscle cells. It is the coordination with respect to time and site that permits blood, after being collected in the atria, to be pumped into the ventricles and to be pressed toward the arteries. To allow coordination, the heart is provided with an **excitation propagation system:** After the atria contract, nerve fibers pick up the excitation and conduct it across an electrically insulating barrier to the top of the heart, from where it is disseminated over the ventricular muscle cells according to the domino principle, thus allowing the ventricular muscle to press from the top toward the blood outlet at the bottom of the heart. After the heartbeat, muscle cells recover and again

reach their steady state, awaiting the next excitation.

Because of these three properties, the heart is able to continue pumping as long as everything happens as it should and as long as the heart muscle cells pass on their excitations in the proper direction. The weak point in this system is that as soon as the muscle cells have recovered from excitation, there is some danger that they may be excited again for some reason. In this case, however, it cannot be foreseen in which direction they will pass on their excitation, so coordination may be disrupted.

4. *Increased recovery period:* To recover from excitation, heart muscle cells need 100-fold the time required by nerve cells. This **increased recovery period** assures that the excitation front has gone sufficiently far before the cells that were just excited regain their excitability. This prevents reexcitations and assures the coordination and reliability of the heart's action.

The short duration, however, from total excitation to steady state remains the Achilles' heel of the heart: If in this phase a further excitation is released (e.g., by external causes like an electric current), coordination breaks down at the moment when muscle cells of different regions of the heart are in different states of excitation. Therefore, by chance, these cells may be stimulated again, the excitation of which has diminished just sufficiently to allow them to be reexcited; instead of doing coordinated pumping, the heart muscle begins to tremble. As a consequence, blood circulation breaks down.

Because the heart is not able to regain coordinated excitation without external help (defibrillation), this situation is extremely dangerous. An electrocardiogram shows this condition by a change from the periodic signals to spiky signals with weaker amplitudes (Figure 4.2).

4.3 From Perception to Danger

Perhaps you have heard the advice not to lie down on the ground during thunderstorms, but to try to squat with the legs together. The disadvantage arising from being a more exposed target for lightning is offset by the benefit of increased protection of the heart: If lightning does not strike one directly but only hits the earth nearby, a part of the lightning current will follow the roundabout way across the body. Because our body is a good electrical conductor, once the current enters the body, it is spread over the entire internal region,

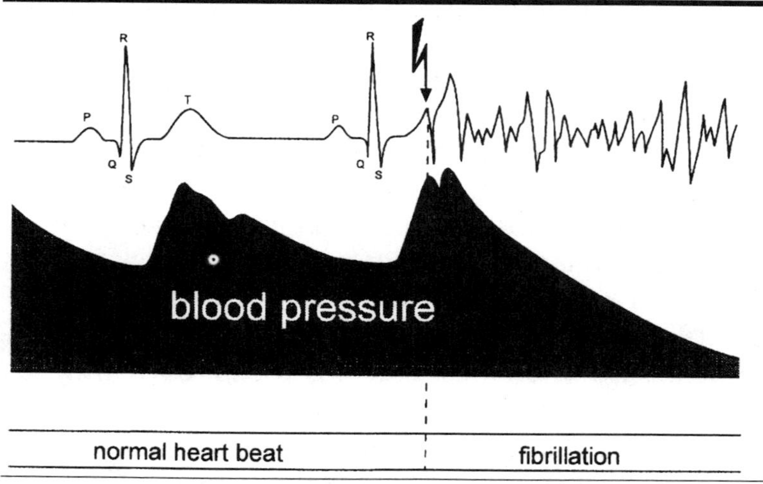

Figure 4.2. Electrocardiogram and blood pressure recordings during heart fibrillation.

although with different concentrations: Blood vessels and muscles are preferred; fat and bone are avoided. It is the amount of current flowing across the heart that determines the risk. This, in turn, is dependent on the current entrance and exit points. The least hazardous case is when the current flows from one foot to the other, because then the heart is lying considerably aside, with the effect that only 7 percent of the current follows the roundabout way across the heart.

The most common type of electrical accident occurs under single-fault conditions in which one hand touches a live part and the failure current longitudinally flows across the body to the grounded feet. This type of case is commonly referred to if current amplitudes are related to biological effects. It is, however, not the most dangerous one: The worst case is to touch a live part with one hand, while the other hand is simultaneously in contact with a grounded part (e.g., another device). In this case danger occurs even at one-third lower current amplitudes. To sit on a defective heating blanket and to touch the grounded bedpost is less dangerous and requires currents with a 40 percent higher amplitude than in the longitudinal reference case (Table 4.1). If not otherwise indicated in this book, the given electric current amplitudes refer to the longitudinal flow from hands to feet.

4.3.1 Direct Current Effects

Direct currents cannot excite cells. Therefore, they are less dangerous than sinusoidal currents. At longitudinal current pathways direct currents must exceed **2 mA** to be perceived (e.g., a feeling of warmth or a weak tingling). With increasing current amplitude the sensation is intensified and eventually changes to pain.

Current Entrance	Current Exit	
	Left Hand	Right Hand
Foot (feet)	1.0	0.8
Other hand	0.4	0.4
Back	0.7	0.3
Seat	0.7	0.7
Chest	1.5	1.3

Table 4.1. Conversion Factors for Different Current Pathways to Obtain Equivalent Amplitudes to Cause Heart Fibrillation (Sam 1969)

Above **40 mA,** currents disturb the excitation propagation. This diminishes after switch-off but becomes dangerous if the action of the heart is disturbed to such a degree that fibrillation takes place, which must be considered over **150 mA,** provided the duration exceeds the period of a heartbeat. Shorter intervals are less critical. The fibrillation threshold is increased to **500 mA** if the duration is less than 10 percent of the heartbeat period.

Direct current hazards depend on the current flow direction as well. Near the cathode the excess of negatively charged particles reduces the excitation threshold and makes cells more sensitive to external stimuli. For regions near the positive pole, the opposite applies: The increase of the surplus of positive electric charges makes cells less sensitive to external stimuli. Because of the reduction of the heart's excitation threshold, pathways with the negative pole near the heart increase the probability of fibrillation and, therefore, are more dangerous.

In spite of the fact that direct currents are less dangerous, small amplitudes may not be negligible. The reason lies in the current's property of not changing with time. In sinusoidal currents, due to the continuous change of flow direction, electric charges essentially oscillate around their position, whereas DC charges continue to move in the same direction (which is different for charges with different polarity). Charges are separated from each other and transported toward the counterpoles (electrolysis). This results in accumulations at the contact areas (e.g., of [positive] hydrogen ions at the [negative] cathode and of [negative] hydroxide ions at the [positive] anode).

In medical technology this property is ambivalent: Its benefit lies in the fact that direct currents can be used to transport drugs and pharmaceuticals across the skin into the body (iontophoresis). The disadvantage is that at the contact areas the accumulation of ions may lead to chemical reactions and to tissue cauterization and inflammation. This is especially critical at active electric implants: They are fed by batteries, and as they may remain inside the body for many years, unavoidable DC leakage currents, which may be negligible under conditions of transient use, may cause complications. This is why, for implantable pacemakers, the limit values for DC leakage currents are decreased to 0.1 mA, which is only 1 percent of the lowest limit for sinusoidal currents.

In high tension accidents and, of course, also in direct lightning strikes, transcorporal currents can exceed 10 A. Such high values can cause internal burns, mainly at the joints. A summary of the dependence of biological effects on DC amplitude and duration is given in Figure 4.3.

4.3.2 Mains Frequency Current Effects

Mains frequency sinusoidal currents can fulfill all three requirements for stimulation (duration, speed of change, and amplitude). They can excite cells and, therefore, are biologically more efficient than direct currents. If their amplitude exceeds the perception threshold, they are perceived as tingling, pulling, or scarifying. Longitudinal pathway currents of only **0.5 mA** are perceived. This is only a quarter of the equivalent DC value. With increasing amplitude the sensation is intensified, the number of excited muscle cells is increased, and the muscle begins to cramp.

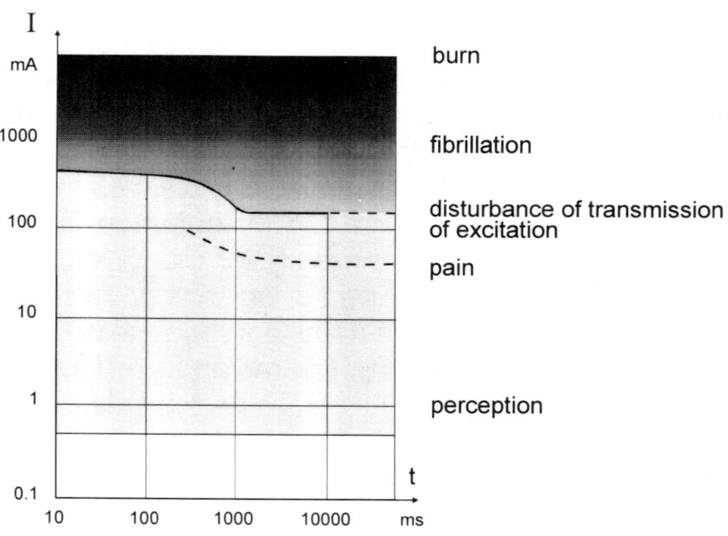

Figure 4.3. DC bioeffects depending on amplitude and duration.

Danger arises if cramping of the hand becomes so strong that it is impossible to release a touched live object by one's own will. The amplitude that causes this reaction is called the *let-go threshold.* It differs from person to person. For safety considerations it is assumed to be **10 mA.** If the current amplitude is further increased, the breathing muscles are also affected: At longer durations, breathing is impaired, with danger of suffocation.

At **40 mA** 95 percent of persons will have heart fibrillation if the duration exceeds several heartbeats. In case of contact times shorter than 10 percent of a heartbeat interval, the fibrillation threshold is increased up to the fourfold amplitude (Figure 4.4). The

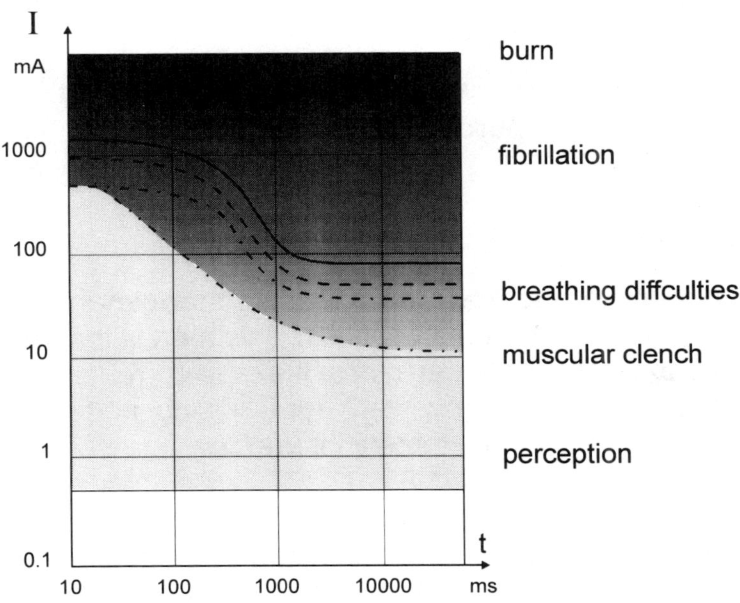

Figure 4.4. Mains frequency AC bioeffects depending on amplitude and duration.

lower hazard at short durations has an important consequence for safety precautions. To make use of this advantage, circuit breakers, especially residual current protective devices, must be constructed so as to switch off the circuit in a sufficiently short time (i.e., 0.2–0.5 seconds).

Biological current effects can be summarized as follows:

Short durations are fourfold less dangerous!

**Alternating currents are fourfold
more dangerous than direct currents!**

**Danger thresholds exceed perception
thresholds by 10-fold!**

**Danger to life begins above the 100-fold
perception threshold!**

4.4 Safe Current Limits

In principle, there are no materials that can insulate live parts ideally (see chapter 3). This means that even with extensive effort, electrical leakage currents of devices cannot be prevented from flowing across the body, if one touches the enclosure.

Because it is not possible to avoid leakage currents, safety standards limit their amplitudes based on worst-case assumptions, namely, that an electrically conducting person with impaired protection of the skin who is ideally connected to the ground touches the enclosure of a device. This provides an additional safety margin because, in practice, there are several resistances in effect that further limit current flow (skin resistance, shoe resistance, ground resistance). The values agreed on reflect the compromise between cost and benefit (see chapter 1).

In daily life where **household devices** are used, safety considerations can be restricted to short-term contacts with the enclosure of a device only. It is, therefore, sufficient to define limit values for *enclosure leakage currents* to prevent danger. For permanently installed devices, such as washing machines, the safety factor is only three (according to EN 60335-1 the *device leakage current* is allowed to reach 3.5 mA). The reason is that in this case perception can be accepted, and even to startle back does not pose further risk. For handheld devices, such as drills or mixers, the limit is lower; **0.25 mA** has been chosen to avoid perception and possible shock reactions under normal conditions.

Electromedical devices must have improved insulation from mains voltage. This is reflected by lower leakage current values and has several rationales:

1. Shock reactions may result in uncontrolled movements that in a sensible environment, like in an operation theatre, can lead to fatal consequences.

2. Leakage currents may be introduced into the patient's body if the user simultaneously is in contact with the patient and the enclosure of a device (Figure 4.5).

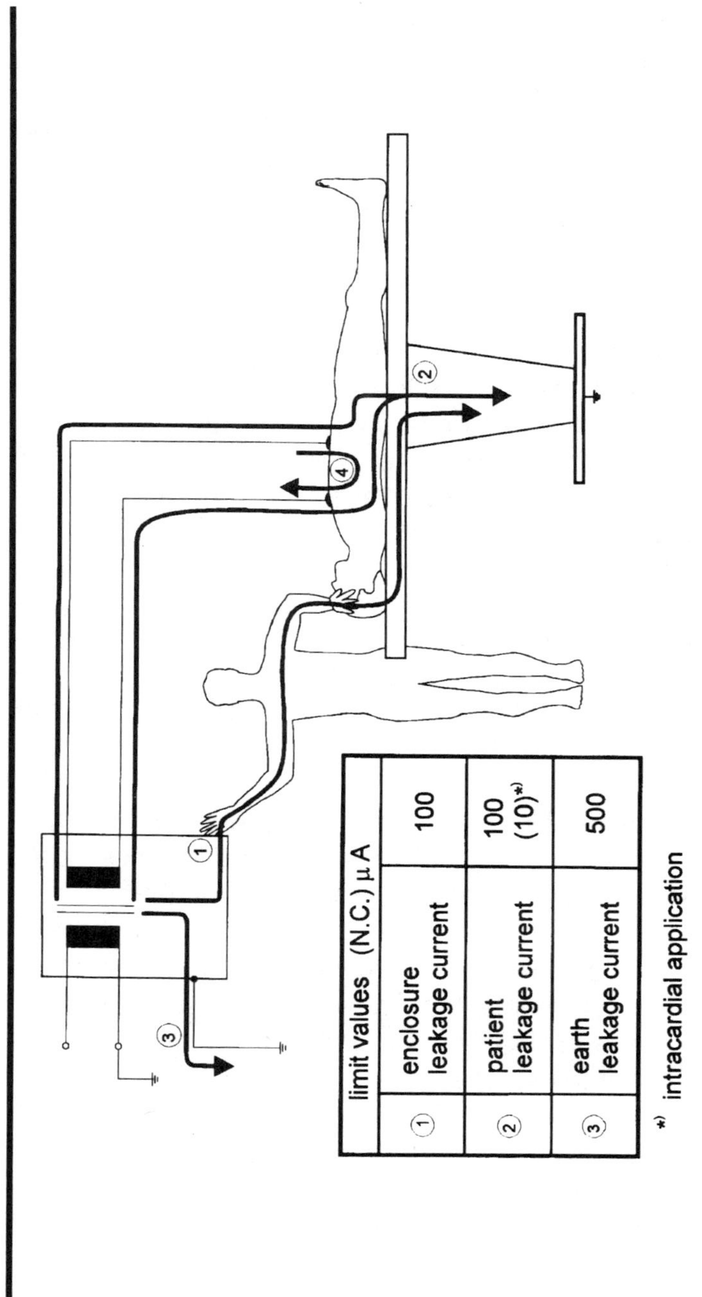

Figure 4.5. Possible leakage currents of electromedical devices.

3.   In contrast to household devices, electro-medical devices may have applied parts that are intended to come in contact with the patient or his internal organs for a long time (lung ventilators, electrocardiogram monitors, suction devices). Therefore, leakage currents from applied parts (*patient leakage currents*), especially if used in the open heart, require increased attention. Examples are active electrodes for high frequency surgery devices, ultrasound transducers for intrasurgical investigation of the heart, and angiographic catheters, which are introduced at peripheral arteries and pushed forward to the heart.

4.   As applied parts may come into direct contact with the patient's organs, there is no additional safety margin provided by additional electrical resistances.

The limits for *enclosure leakage currents* and *patient leakage currents* are both **0.1 mA** and lie below the perception threshold by a factor of five. Patient leakage currents of applied parts for cardiac application (CF type applied parts) are reduced by one magnitude and amount to **0.01 mA.** Although reduced, this value is a compromise. Because they are applied directly to the heart, currents of 0.1 mA can cause fibrillation in 50 percent of patients. If the usual safety factor of two magnitudes to the danger limit was applied, this would require patient leakage currents as low as 0.001 mA, which cannot be reasonably achieved; therefore, a safety factor of 10 must be accepted. This means that even if the devices meet the requirement, patient leakage currents of 0.01 mA still have a fibrillation probability of 1:500. Because of this smaller safety margin, an excess of patient leakage currents for CF applied parts must be considered especially critical.

Excess of CF patient leakage currents should not be tolerated!

So far, our considerations have been based on the bio-effects of leakage currents. However, there is another aspect that must be considered as well. On the one hand, leakage currents flowing across the insulation to grounded parts cannot be biologically significant, because they are flowing along the protective earth lead to the ground (*earth leakage currents*). On the other hand, there are good reasons to limit these currents as well: First, earth leakage currents are additive if many devices are in operation; the protective earth lead would have to carry considerable amounts of currents. The consequence is that these currents may cause potential differences that might be no longer negligible (see also chapter 7). Second, mains cables are frequently moved. This puts the protective earth lead at considerable risk of breaking, resulting in a single-fault condition in which the earth leakage current must flow along another path to the ground. In fact, it would add to the enclosure leakage current and might become relevant for the patient. For these reasons, the earth leakage current is limited as well, with a maximum permissible amplitude of **0.5 mA** in normal condition.

4.4.1 Multiple Socket Outlets

If any device is connected by its own mains cable to a fixed, installed, mains socket outlet, it is improbable that the protective earth lead will break in more than one mains cable at once. However, if a flexible multiple socket outlet is used, which, for instance, supplies five devices, the protective earth lead interruption of the common mains cable becomes more important: In this case the earth leakage currents of all five devices would add to the enclosure leakage current of any of these devices. Under worst-case conditions this could result in an excess of the enclosure leakage current by 26-fold (5 × 0.5 mA + 0.1 mA). Even the limit for a single-fault condition would be exceeded by fivefold. Such currents already lie above the perception threshold. Therefore, it is recommended that flexible multiple socket outlets not be used.

Avoid flexible multiple socket outlets!

Anyone who has seen operation theatres in use knows that this recommendation is rarely observed. These locations are characterized by the increased use of medical electrical devices. Therefore, the number of fixed, installed, mains socket outlets soon proves to be inadequate. In such cases the construction of permanently installed ceiling hangings would be the best solution.

If the use of flexible multiple socket outlets is unavoidable, risks can be reduced by additional means. The simplest one is not to connect more than one protectively earthed device: Double-insulated devices do not pose this problem because of the missing connection to the earth. A further possibility is to use a common mains cable with deliberately oversized cross sections to reduce the probability of a protective earth lead interruption. A further way to reduce risk is to place the multiple socket outlet in such a location that the mains cable is protected from mechanical stress as much as possible. These recommendations can be summarized as follows:

Prefer connection of double-insulated devices!

Protect the mains cable from mechanical stress!

Use an oversized mains cable!

In addition, the use of flexible multiple socket outlets has two additional disadvantages:

1. The possibility of multiplying the number of connected devices at the same electrical circuit increases the overload probability. If the overcurrent protection device is activated, many devices, even life-supporting ones, would fail at once.

2. The next problem arises in explosive zones, which in operation theatres are assumed to be on the floor. If a multiple socket outlet is lying on the floor, there is some probability of stumbling over one of the mains cables and accidentally pulling out the mains plug. Under usual conditions this would have no further consequences besides the unintentional disconnecting of a device and perhaps losing one's balance and falling down. Flammable mixtures (e.g., of disinfectants or anaesthetic gases), even with burn-promoting gases, are heavier than air. These gases might accumulate on the floor. The disconnection of the mains plug may cause an electric interruption spark in this critical region and may cause the flammable mixtures to ignite.

For these reasons flexible multiple socket outlets must not lie on the floor! (Extension cables for a single device are prohibited in any case; if the mains cable of a device proves to be too short, it must be replaced by a longer one!)

Do not lay multiple socket outlets on the floor!

4.5 Safe Voltage Limits

For safety considerations a knowledge of the biological effects of electric currents is very important. It is the basis for deriving safety limits for leakage currents. In fact, the measurement of leakage currents allows us to assess the status of electrical insulation and to detect dangerous deteriorations before they can cause accidents.

In daily life, however, it is essential to become aware of hazards without preventive measurements. We already know that electric voltages determine the hazard potential (see chapter 3), but we have also learned that other circumstances may play a major role. We have seen that nerve cells can be excited if exposed to voltages of only 20 mV; yet our children are allowed to play with electric toy trains and to touch 1000-fold higher voltages (12 V) without any hazard. The reason for this is the electrical resistance of our body, which determines whether a contact with live parts will result in a dangerous current flow.

4.5.1 The Body's Electrical Resistance

The assessment of the body's electrical resistance started at the beginning of the 20th century, first by studying dead bodies. To clarify whether these results were also valid for living persons, it was necessary to also make measurements on volunteers (Biegelmeier 1986). Today, we know that the body's resistance is not only determined by intracorporal electrical conductivity, but that our skin also plays an important role in protecting against electrical hazards and contributes significantly to the total body resistance (Figure 4.6).

**body resistance =
skin resistance + intracorporal resistance**

Of course, the effective body resistance is dependent on the pathway of the electric current. If flowing from hand to hand, it amounts to 2000 Ω, with similar contributions from the skin and the intracorporal region.

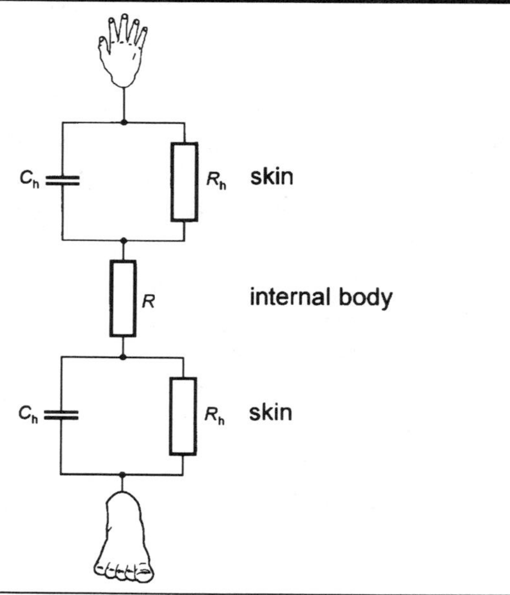

Figure 4.6. Equivalent diagram for electrical body resistance.

The **skin,** especially its dry outer layer, is responsible for the frequency dependence of body resistance: From mains frequency down to direct currents, it increases almost to the doubled value. In addition, the electrical body resistance is voltage dependent. This is because voltage amplitudes below 75 V are too small to allow a breakthrough across the outer layer of the skin.

Special attention is necessary if the insulating properties of our skin are impaired or even missing. This is the case, for example, with wet hands or at wounds. Wearing (insulating) surgical gloves also provides electrical protection, which is especially important when using high frequency surgery.

In a single-fault condition it is more dangerous to hold a portable device or an applied part than to touch a live part of standing equipment. The reason is that the protective skin resistance is reduced with the increase of the contact area and contact pressure.

The **internal body resistance,** except in the high frequency range, is dependent neither on voltage nor on frequency. As bone is a poor conductor, electrical resistance is dependent mainly on the cross section of soft tissues: Resistance increases with a decrease in the cross-sectional area. In this respect the most unfavorable conditions can be found at the joints, especially at the ankles; these in turn contribute most to the value of internal body resistance. As the heating caused by electric currents increases with resistance, it is not surprising that joints, in particular, are injured at currents higher than 10 A (Figure 4.7).

Internal electrical body resistance is dependent on the electric current pathway across the body. In most

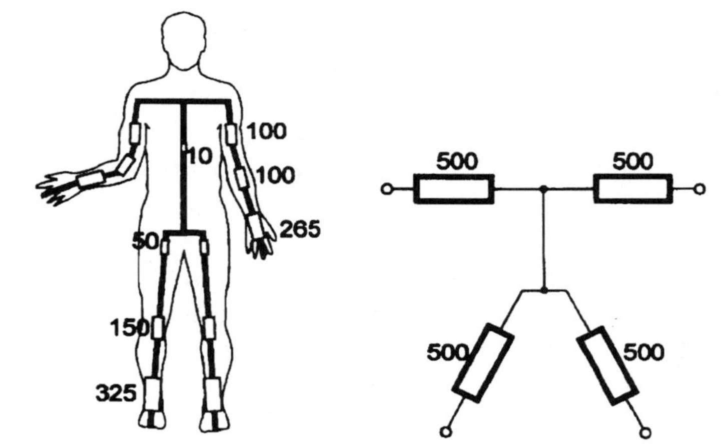

Figure 4.7. Distribution of internal body resistance and a simplified equivalent diagram.

cases, it is sufficient to approximate the situation by representing each extremity by a 500 Ω resistance. Thus, the internal body resistance for a hand-hand pathway is 1000 Ω. In the case of a current flow from one hand to both grounded feet, the internal resistance is reduced to 750 Ω. If the second hand touches the live part as well, the current flows from both hands to both feet, and the internal resistance is further reduced to only 500 Ω.

4.5.2 Dangerous Voltages

With this knowledge we are now able to derive values of dangerous voltages by applying the fundamental law of electrotechnology (**voltage = current × resistance,** chapter 3). Figure 4.8 shows the result: If current amplitudes with known bioeffects are multiplied by the relevant body resistance, one obtains the related

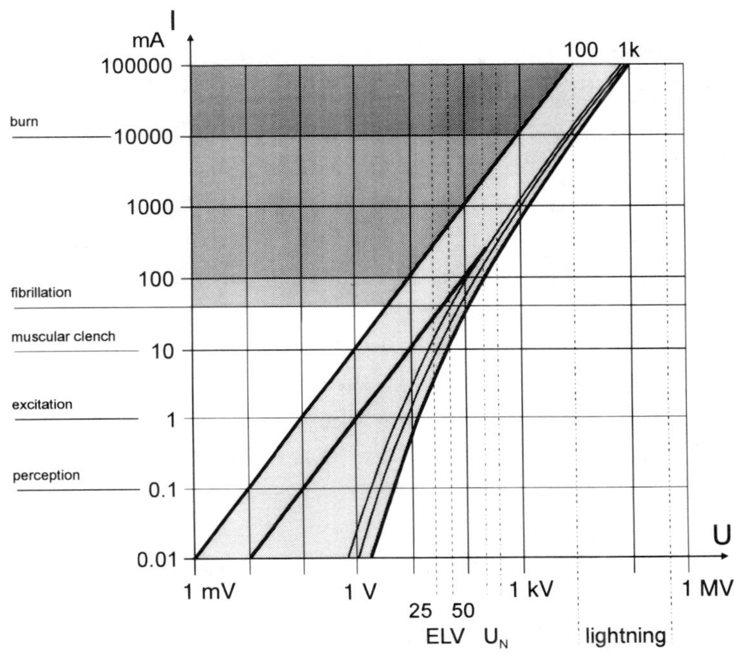

Figure 4.8. Current-voltage relationship when in contact with live parts.

voltages. Therefore, two cases can be differentiated: The one of intact skin with higher body resistances, and the other with reduced body resistance (e.g., for patients during surgical treatments).

In the case of **intact skin** (body resistance = 2000 Ω), the American mains voltage (see Figure 3.2) approaches the fibrillation threshold. The European mains voltage is high enough to cause heart fibrillation (Figure 4.8). The voltage that is equivalent to the "let-go threshold" is 50 V. In general, the effective resistance is higher because of the protective effect of additional resistances that must be taken into account (resistance of shoes and grounding conditions). This explains why there is an additional safety margin that allows **50 V** to be considered without danger in daily life. It is, therefore, defined as general *safety extra low voltage* (SELV). In the medical field this value is reduced by a factor of two to **25 V,** which constitutes the *medical safety extra low voltage* (MSELV) for mains frequency.

As DC voltages are less dangerous, the corresponding values can be higher and are **120 V** for general DC SELV in daily life and **60 V** in a medical environment for DC MSELV.

MSELVs are 25 V (50/60 Hz) and 60 V (DC)

If the protective effect of the **skin is missing,** as is the case with wounds or during surgical operations, the effective resistance is much lower and reduced to the intracorporal resistance. Depending on the current pathway, it may lie in the range of about 100 Ω to 1000 Ω. In these situations even contact with MSELVs could be dangerous. This is why, in contrast to household devices, the use of SELV is not accepted as additional safety means for medical electrical devices!

From Figure 4.8 it follows that for body resistances of 100 Ω, the let-go current corresponds to voltages of only **1 V!** In operation theatres it is necessary to avoid even the appearance of such low voltages. Even more critical are surgical treatments or investigations that need direct contact with the heart. To guard against hazards even in such circumstances, voltages as low as **10 mV** should be avoided. Such low voltages are not uncommon, whether in daily life or within hospitals. They may be measured between devices that are connected to different electric circuits, between parts of a medical system, or even between accessible parts of a single device. Therefore, additional potential equilibration is required.

4.6 Common Voltage Sources

In daily life accessible electrical voltages are encountered more frequently than perhaps many of us may be aware. **DC voltages** are present not only in batteries, where they usually range from 1.5 V to 12 V, but in each separation of materials (e.g., when rising from a chair); each rubbing of two objects (e.g., when combing freshly washed hair or putting on a pullover); each movement causing separation of electrical charges and as a consequence the appearance of DC electric voltages (chapter 3). These voltages can even be high enough to exceed the insulation property of air and may lead to perceptible spark discharges.

Electrostatic charging requires the presence of at least one poorly conducting material, such as woolen clothing, supported by low air humidity. Accordingly, it can be avoided by increasing air humidity and the conductivity of objects. In operation theatres this is done not only to prevent annoying microshocks but also the ignition of flammable mixtures by spark discharges. Electrostatic charging can be reduced by providing clothes with at least 30 percent cotton content, using air humidifiers, installing electrically conducting floors, and grounding insulated metal parts, such as trolleys or device holders. For this reason, mobile devices must have conducting wheels if they are intended for use in operation theatres.

Alternating voltages may occur in other situations besides single-fault conditions. Much more frequent are voltages caused by the flow of (leakage) currents across resistances. An earth leakage current of 0.5 mA may cause a voltage of 0.1 mV between the device enclosure and the mains plug if the protective earth resistance amounts to 0.2 Ω (which is still in accordance with the requirements). In general, this can be neglected. However, if earth leakage currents are additive in the protective earth leads of the installation, voltage differences of several volts may be measured between devices if they are connected to socket outlets of different electric circuits or in extended medical systems in different rooms.

In addition, it must be taken into account that different electrical conducting parts may exhibit different electric potentials. This can be caused by electric fields, which are omnipresent in our environment. The resulting electric voltages depend on the geometric relations of the metallic parts to each other and to the field source (capacitive coupling).

4.6.1 Potential Equalization

Special potential equalization is necessary in zones where voltages as low as 1 V (in intensive care units and in operation theatres for general surgery) or even 10 mV (in operation theatres for cardiac treatment) are possibly dangerous.

Such low voltages cannot be avoided by device technology alone; additional precautions are needed, possibly comprising constructional and installational means as well as the cooperation of the medical staff, which must care for additional potential equalization connections between the devices and installation (chapter 7). Therefore, yellow/green cables for potential equalization should be available, and medical staff should use them to connect devices with the relevant terminal points at the walls.

According to EN 60601-1-1, the zone where such additional precautions must be taken is the patient's environment, which ranges up to a distance of 1.5 m from the intended position of the patient for diagnostic or therapeutic treatment (Figure 4.9).

Potential equalization cables must be used!

4.7 Safety Precautions

So far, it has been shown that currents less than 2 percent of those that flow through a 100 W bulb may be dangerous. To reduce risk to an acceptable level, safety precautions are necessary. As already mentioned, the design of electrical equipment must assure **double protection;** that is, two equivalent safety means must be available and must be independent of each other to assure protection even under single-fault conditions (see chapter 1). In medical device technology one must at least be prevented from touching any live part (except if it is assured that currents will not exceed the leakage current limits).

4.7.1 Basic Insulation

The most important safety precaution is to surround accessible live parts with protective insulation (basic insulation). It must be assured that this insulation is preserved throughout the device's lifetime. This means that insulation material is allowed neither to be impaired with age nor to exhibit safety-relevant changes

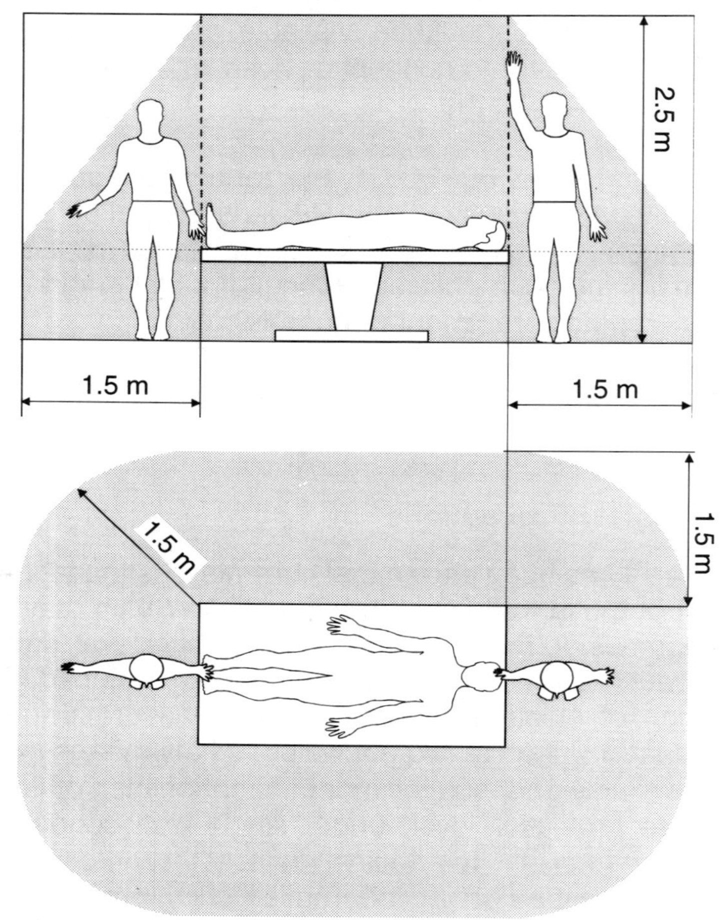

Figure 4.9. Patient environment (where additional safety precautions are needed).

due to forseeable influences, such as thermal or chemical stress.

However, not all common materials meet this requirement. Even the most widely used insulation material,

PVC, is for restricted application only. If heated to more than 75°C, it becomes inflexible and if moved, full of rents. As certain parts within devices are allowed to reach considerably higher temperatures, the proper internal wiring of devices is important to avoid thermal overexposure. For instance, transformers, even under normal conditions, are allowed to reach temperatures up to 180°C if insulated with adequate material!

Plastic enclosures may become inflexible and may lose their resistance to impact if exposed to thermal and chemical stress. An ultrasonic company learned this after transducers produced by the company were frequently complained about because of rents in the enclosures. It turned out that the plastic material was not sufficiently resistant to the disinfectants used and, therefore, its mechanical properties had changed with time.

In addition, there exists material (e.g., natural rubber) that may be impaired with time even without any external influence. Over the years it may become full of rents, lose its mechanical stability, and finally become detached from the live part.

Wood should be avoided for several reasons. It changes its insulating property with humidity and increases the hazard of burns. For household devices wooden enclosures are permitted as long as they are not responsible for insulation. Other insulation materials that are not suited for protective insulation include casting compounds that deform with heat.

4.7.2 Functional Insulation

Insulation that is not intended for safety but only for maintaining the function (*functional insulation*) does not need to fulfill such rigorous requirements. Thus, even varnish can be accepted (as done for transformer windings).

4.7.3 Medical Device Safety Strategies

With regard to the additional protection required for medical device technology, (only) three approaches are permitted:

Battery Devices

The most effective protection is to not allow dangerous situations to exist. This is done when designing battery-driven devices. They do not need to be connected to the dangerous mains voltage or with earth potential and, therefore, may be an effective solution if these devices do not produce dangerous voltages.

Choosing which devices can be battery driven sometimes cannot be determined easily. Many devices (such as defibrillators) can be operated either with a mains power supply or by their internal batteries. The pure existence of a mains plug, however, is not sufficient to conclude that such a battery device is not protected according to the battery device philosophy. The point is whether the device can still be operated as intended once it is connected to the mains voltage. If the intended use is prevented during mains connection by design (e.g., by a movable cover that allows access either to the mains plug or the patient outlets only), it can be considered a battery device. But if the intended use is still possible after connection to the mains voltage, the device must be protected either by protective earthing or by double insulation.

A frequent problem with battery devices is the connection of the electric circuits of the applied part with the metallic enclosure. When such connections exist, it is possible that the patient will be exposed to external voltages, such as electrostatic potentials or potential differences. Electric circuits of applied parts must be insulated from accessible conducting parts of the enclosure.

Double Insulation (Safety Class II)

Double insulation is based on the provision of two equivalent insulations—the basic insulation and an additional insulation. This principle is applied, for instance, at mains cords. The advantage is that protection is not dependent on further external conditions. This is why most handheld household devices (except electric irons) or handheld electric tools use this means of protection. It can be identified by the protection class label, which consists of two concentric squares (see Figure 5.4) and by the (flat) two-pin mains plug.

The advantage of being independent of further external protective means is offset by a significant disadvantage: The single-fault condition is no longer indicated and continues to be present. Thus, from that time on only single protection is provided. The probability of an insulation failure is not small; it can be estimated to be 1:100.

Double-insulated devices, therefore, inherently require periodic inspection of the insulation. However, it must be emphasized that regular safety tests with intervals of one to three years cannot replace routine visual inspection by the user. Damage to the insulation must not be tolerated and must be treated seriously and competently. Adhesive strips are not adequate electrical insulation material. On the contrary, they are produced so as to have a pH value equivalent to that of the wound and to be permeable by humidity; unfortunately, they are permeable by electric currents as well.

Safety class II inherently requires periodic inspection!

Electric insulation requires frequent inspection by the user!

Insulation damages are dangerous and must not be tolerated!

Adhesive strips are not adequate for electrical insulation!

Protective Earthing (Safety Class I)

Everyone has likely experienced a blown fuse and an interrupted electric circuit as a result of an insulation failure. This great advantage of indicating the single-fault condition and switching off the electric voltage must be weighed against a disadvantage: Protection is provided if not only the device itself but also the electrical installation meet the safety requirements. To be able to understand this, we must consider the single-fault situation in more detail.

The *initial situation:* In general, our electric power supply is based on grounded nets, which means that one of the two leads (the blue insulated "neutral lead") is connected to the ground, whereas the second "live" one presents a voltage relative to the ground (e.g., of 230 V [mains voltage]). In the distribution box electric circuits are protected from overload (e.g., by fuses or by automatic circuit breakers). The protective earth lead is connected to the grounding network of a house with a certain resistance. This resistance partly depends on the cross section and the overall length of the protective earth leads.

The *single-fault situation* (Figure 4.10): If, because of damage to the insulation, a live lead comes in contact with a metallic (earthed) enclosure, it becomes short circuited and a current flows that, according to Ohm's law, is determined by the value of the earth

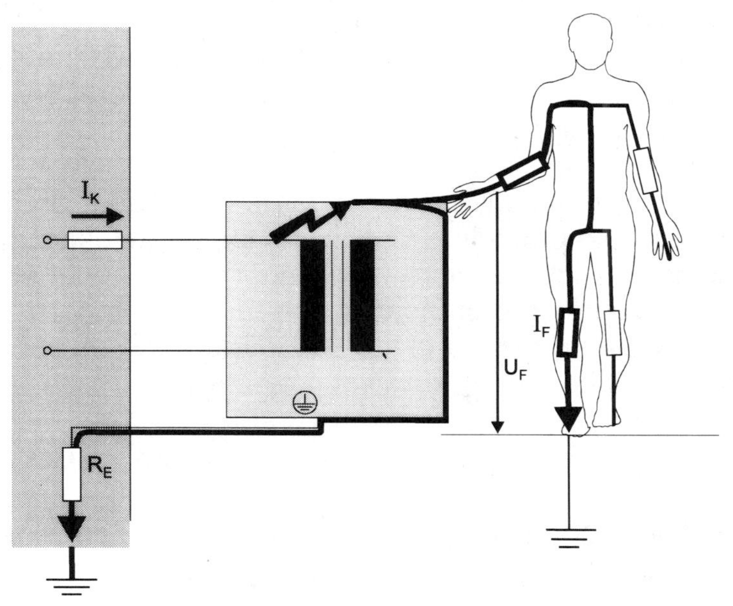

Figure 4.10. Single fault at a protectively earthed device.

resistance. In the first moment the enclosure still exhibits a voltage of 230 V relative to the ground. A usual earth resistance of 0.2 Ω would result in a short-circuit current of 1,150 A! This may result in an overload situation and may even cause a fire. A person who touches the device would still be at risk because of the unreduced voltage. Pure earthing, therefore, is not sufficient for safety. The protection requires further means, namely, overcurrent circuit breakers (fuses) at the installation. They ensure that the electric circuit is interrupted before the short-circuit current can reach its (dangerous) maximum. Depending on the characteristics of the circuit breaker, the switch-off current amplitude usually is limited to five or ten times the nominal current. It is the switch-off current that determines the value of the failure voltage at the device: If the nominal value is 10 A, the switch-off current is five times that, and the earth resistance is 0.2 Ω, the failure voltage would be only 10 V and, therefore, would not cause any danger.

Whether there will be a danger is dependent on the overcurrent protection means and the earth resistance of the installation, which is the most critical parameter. According to the standards, the failure voltage must not exceed the value of the SELV. The following condition must be met for efficient protective earthing:

switch-off current × earth resistance < SELV

Besides earthing conditions, safety depends considerably on circuit breakers as well. Fuses are frequently "repaired" by surrounding the blown one by aluminum foil or by turning around a copper wire. When this is done, however, much higher currents than intended may flow in a short-circuit case. This annuls the protection philosophy and can cause fire and dangerous failure voltages.

Botched fuses cause life and fire hazards!

For protective earthing the requirements on the quality of the grounding net are not easy to meet: For a 16 A electric circuit with a 10-fold switch-off current, the ground resistance of the entire installation should not exceed 0.15 Ω (25 V/160 A). However, the protective earth resistance from the enclosure to the mains plug is already allowed to be 0.2 Ω (for old devices even more). Therefore, this requirement cannot be met without further precautions. The favorite possibility is the reducing the switch-off current without compromising the nominal load of the electric circuit.

Solving this problem requires the installation of a residual current protective device that monitors whether all of the currents flowing toward the electric devices actually return. If this is not the case, insulation failure occurs and the circuit is switched off. In Austria and Germany, for example, such residual current protective devices are mandatory for grounded nets and must switch off the electric circuit if current differences exceed 30 mA. In our example this reduced switch-off current would allow a 5,500-fold higher earth resistance, namely 833 Ω (25 V/0.03 A), which now can be easily realized. In general, the values are much lower than that.

The use of residual current protective devices is a very efficient means, but it is combined with a typical risk: The switching mechanism on which this precaution must rely may lose its movability and, therefore, fail just when needed. It is recommended to check its function at regular intervals (e.g., monthly) to assure its functionality and to maintain its movability.

Defective residual current protective devices endanger the effect of protective earthing!

Residual current protective devices need periodic function checks!

5 Medical Electrical Devices

5.1 Safety Concept

According to safety standard EN 60601-1, **medical electrical devices must be designed such that their *intended use* in normal condition and in *single-fault condition* will not cause any safety hazard to the *user*, the *patient*, or the *environment* that could *be foreseen reasonably* (and that is not inherent in the intended use), provided they are *installed* and *maintained* according to their instructions for use.**

Do not trust the first glance: This general requirement is far from being without problems. As with the small print of a contract, which requires increased attention, each phrase must be considered very carefully.

First of all, the definition of **medical electrical equipment** must be clarified: The criterion is not only patient application for diagnosis or therapy. Were it so, all sun lamps or muscle stimulators for home use would fall into this group as well. In fact, only those devices that are applied by medical personnel or under their supervision are addressed. This restriction has three different consequences: (1) It can be assumed that the device will be used with care and competence. (2) It cannot be excluded that it might be used on patients who are unconscious or unable to react. (3) It might possibly be used together with other devices and, perhaps, for long-term applications. In contrast, household devices can be assumed to be applied by persons who feel well enough not to go into a hospital and are at least conscious and able to perceive and react. However, it must be taken into account that users might be neither attentive nor careful. These different circumstances must be taken into account by different design strategies and requirements for the devices.

As they differ from other groups of devices, it is important to give the user the chance to identify medical electrical devices easily. First of all, this is provided by the manufacturer's definition of the intended use that must be contained in the instructions for use. Second, there must be markings on the devices with symbols that at the same time indicate that the insulation of the applied part(s) belongs to one of three types (Figure 5.1):

- **Type B** electromedical devices that either need no contact with the patient at all (e.g., infrared radiation devices, laser therapy equipment, ultrasound nebulizers) or for which the applied part is protectively earthed.

- **Type BF** electromedical devices that have an applied part that is insulated from the earth (floating) (e.g., nerve and muscle stimulators, infusion pumps, high frequency surgical devices).

- **Type CF** electromedical devices that have an applied part that is intended for cardiac application. It not only is insulated from earth (floating) but is also characterized by an

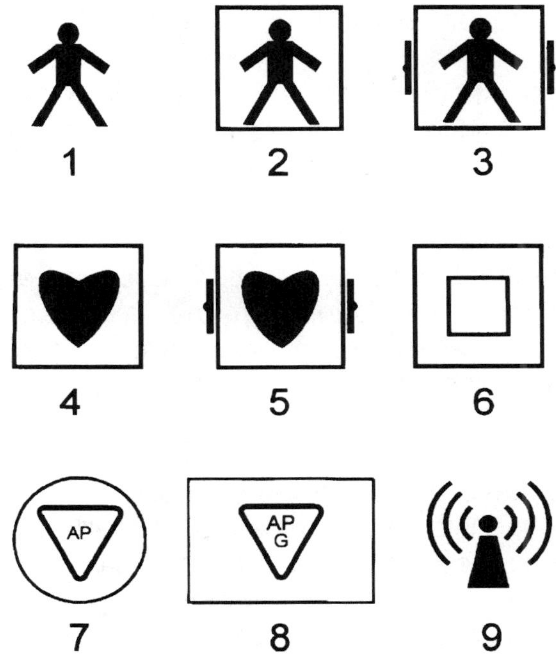

Figure 5.1. Symbols for the classification of devices: 1—electromedical device type B. If there is an applied part, it is portectively earthed (in future: applied part type B connected to the earth); 2—electromedical device type BF with a floating applied part (in future: applied part type BF insulated from the earth); 3—electromedical device type BF protected against the influence of defibrillators; 4—electromedical device type CF with floating applied part for cardiac use (in future: applied part type CF for cardiac use); 5—electromedical device type CF protected against the influence of defibrillators; 6—double-insulated device (protection class II); 7—explosion proof device for mixtures with air (chapter 6); 8—explosion proof device for mixtures with oxygen (chapter 6); 9—device with intended emission of nonionizing radiation.

extra low patient leakage current (which re-flects the improved insulation).

The amendment to IEC 601-1/1995, which has not yet been adopted in Europe, has changed the meaning of the type groups and has restricted it to applied parts only. In the future we will speak of applied parts as type B, BF, or CF only. Devices are permitted to carry all three symbols, provided their applied parts differ with respect to insulation from the earth (e.g., patient monitors, ultrasonic scanners with electrocardiogram trigger facilities, and defibrillators with integrated electrocardiogram monitors).

It has already been mentioned that the manufacturer is not responsible for eliminating all possible hazards, only those that are combined with the **intended use.** It is not the *actual* use that, for instance, makes a hair cutter a medical device—just because the head of a patient is prepared for brain surgery. The intended use is defined only by the manufacturer who classifies his product (e.g., an ultraviolet radiation device is either a household device or it is medical electrical equipment). Therefore, the manufacturer is allowed not to make a foot switch watertight if its application within operation theatres is excluded.

The reference to the device's intended use, however, means that the user is charged with responsibility, because he is assumed to be familiar with the device—its method of application and its instructions for use.

Depending on the point of view, the fact that safety precautions must also be taken into account for single-fault conditions can be seen positively or negatively: On the one hand, the principle of double protection might be appreciated. On the other hand, there may be concerns that hazards arising due to further simultaneous faults may not be prevented. What is considered a single fault, however, must be seen very generally: namely, the failure of any safety-relevant part, which may or may not be electrical, or even the occurrence of any abnormal condition.

Protection must be assured under any abnormal condition!

Examples of single-fault conditions are the interruption of the protective earth conductor; the interruption of an active conductor in the mains cable; any insulation failure; a failure of any safety-relevant component (e.g., for current or voltage limitation or for mounting the device); the overload of transformers, heating elements, or motors; an excess of the intended operation time (if not intended for continuous use); the blocking of movable parts (such as ventilators or lifting elements); the impairment of cooling (e.g., by covering cooling slots or the occlusion of filters); the break of a mechanical fixture; the leakage of gas containers or fluid-containing tubes; and spillage, if it could occur during intended use.

Chapter 1 discussed that the effort for precautions is based on a social consensus. The result of cost-benefit considerations is that (only) those hazards that are **reasonably** foreseeable must be prevented. What exactly is understood by this, however, is left open. The final decision probably is reserved for the judgment of a court that might decide case by case. Basically, Murphy's law and the obligation of the manufacturer to perform a risk analysis (e.g., according to EN 1441 [see "Risk Analysis"]), require consideration of all possible failures and assessment of their risk potential. Thus, a device is allowed to be damaged or to break down in a single-fault condition, provided it still remains safe (except that the breakdown as such would possibly pose a harm to the patient).

Risk analysis not only must include common first failure conditions, such as the impairment of insulation due to increased temperature within the device or chemical stress caused by disinfection; it must also include hazards that may arise from the intended function. For instance, it is foreseeable that the side railing of a hospital bed might cause bruises if safety distances are too small or if safety stops are missing. Likewise, it is foreseeable that somebody might push against the protruding piston of a syringe pump and cause the delivery of a dangerous extra dose. If not prevented by design, it is foreseeable that gas connections or battery polarity might be changed by mistake. On the other hand, it is not necessary to protect every device from the ignition of flammable mixtures just because flammable disinfectants *could be* spilled on it.

Devices must not only be safe for patients (which include animals in veterinary medicine as well). The environment must be protected as well. This means that the unintended emission of dangerous substances, radiation, or energy must be prevented by design. Therefore, anaesthetic equipment must not have inadmissible leakages where anaesthetic gas could emerge uncontrollably, X-ray devices must be equipped with radiation protection filters, and laser devices must be provided with shutters that prevent unintended laser emission. In addition, fire protection precautions must be realized (e.g., by avoiding easily flammable material or by preventing excessive temperatures that might lead to the softening or even melting of plastics that could drop out of the device and cause a fire).

The general requirements at the beginning of this chapter allow the identification of three factors on which the safety concept is based:

1. The **manufacturer,** who defines the intended use and the requirements for installation and maintenance, must produce the device according to the technical rules. The manufacturer may observe precautions *as defined by him.* Of course, necessary procedures and maintenance intervals must be included in the instructions for use.

2. The **user,** who must *know* the intended use, is responsible for adequate and competent application.

3. **Hospital management** is responsible for regular maintenance and inspection.

5.2 Risk Analysis

To assure that the product exhibits an acceptable cost-benefit ratio, the manufacturer is obliged to analyze the available information systematically, to identify hazards, and to estimate possible risks of the device (according to EN 1441). The manufacturer must include the risk management file in the technical documentation of the product.

Risk is understood to be the product of occurrence probability and the degree of severity of harm (see chapter 1). Although exact determination is difficult, risk can be at least qualitatively estimated. This is done by classifying **occurrence probability** according to a six-step scale:

- "Frequent"

- "Probable"

- "Occasional"

- "Remote"

- "Improbable"

- "Incredible"

The same is done with the **degree of harm,** which is classified as follows:

- "Negligible harm", with little or even no potential to cause injury

- "Marginal harm", with a certain potential to cause injury

- "Critical harm", with the potential to cause serious injury or death

- "Catastrophic harm", with the potential to cause multiple or serious injuries or deaths

All possible combinations of these groups can be summarized in a risk table (Figure 5.2). Because complete freedom from risk cannot be achieved, the safety concept is based on the valuation of all possible risk

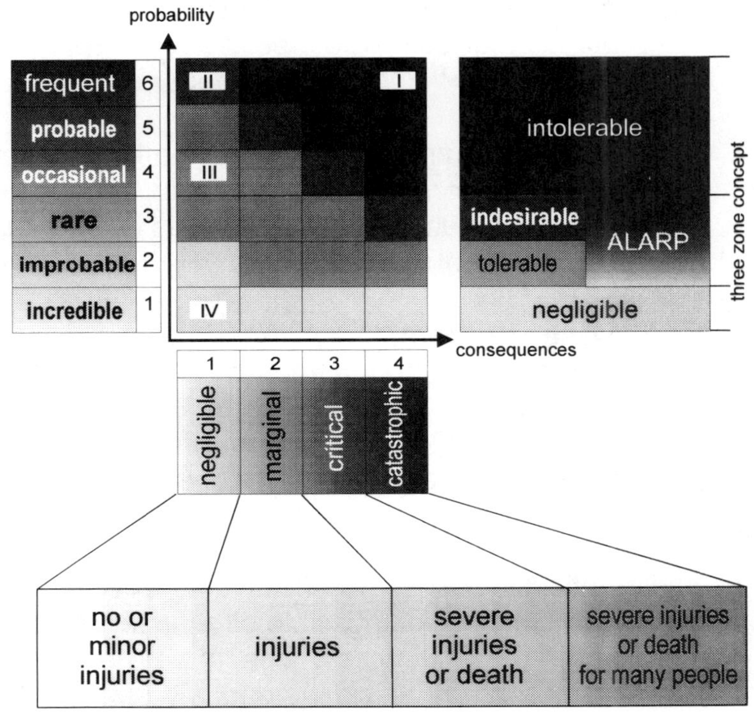

Figure 5.2. Risk table.

groups and the definition of four zones (Note: In zones II and III, risk reduction is oriented to the **ALARP** principle, which means that risk should be **as low as *rea-sonably* p**racticable.):

1. **Zone I** comprises all combinations that are considered to be intolerable risks and that must be excluded.

2. **Zone II** consists of those combinations where risk is undesirable; its avoidance, however, is dependent on cost: Risks in this zone

      are acceptable only if reduction would be impractical or cost would be grossly disproportionate to the improvement gained.

3.   **Zone III** summarizes all combinations where risk reduction would be possible, but where risk can be accepted if cost would exceed the improvement gained.

4.   **Zone IV** comprises those combinations where risk, although improbable, cannot fully be excluded, but where harm, if occurring, is small. Risks in this group are considered negligible or at least tolerable and do not require further actions.

To systematically assess the risks of a device, it is necessary to consider all possible circumstances that may arise from the influences of use, the environment, the interaction with other simultaneously applied devices, and the maintenance requirements, as well as the conditions of production, transport, and storage. For instance, the patient might not be able to react normally because of sickness or drugs or the protective function of the skin might be missing (e.g., in high frequency surgery). In addition, it must be checked whether there are special demands on the reliability or accuracy of the function (e.g., infusion pumps), whether dangerous situations can be recognized (e.g., lasers with invisible light), or whether additional risk factors must be taken into account (e.g., with anaesthetic devices). Risk due to possible human error, especially in stress or emergency situations, must be considered as well.

Starting from a complete function checklist of the device, a list of hazards must be generated. Each hazard must be evaluated and assigned to one of the four risk zones. Depending on the result, it must be established whether the risk can be accepted, by what means (design, conditional precautions, or warnings) risk reduction is possible, and whether the measures taken are effective. After analyzing the entire hazard checklist, it is finally concluded whether the sum of the remaining risks can be accepted or whether the design of the device must be stopped (Figure 5.3).

Risk management is very important, but at the same time it demonstrates what was already pointed out in chapter 1—in spite of the achieved safety level, even for new devices and even in the future, it is not possible to exclude every risk. Therefore, further safety improvements will be possible only through increased knowledge and the conscientiousness of the involved parties.

5.3 Device Identification

It reflects not only politeness but also common sense for two people to introduce themselves at first meeting. Would you have confidence in someone who is completely unknown to you and at whom you did not even look?

In a similar way it makes sense and is important to acquaint yourself with a device (e.g., to clarify whether it is a medical electrical device), and to determine whether it is suited for mains connection in respect to its rated voltage or its nominal current. So, for instance, a device imported from the USA (where mains voltage is only half as high as in Europe) could have a voltage selection means that was adjusted improperly, or high power laser equipment with a nominal current

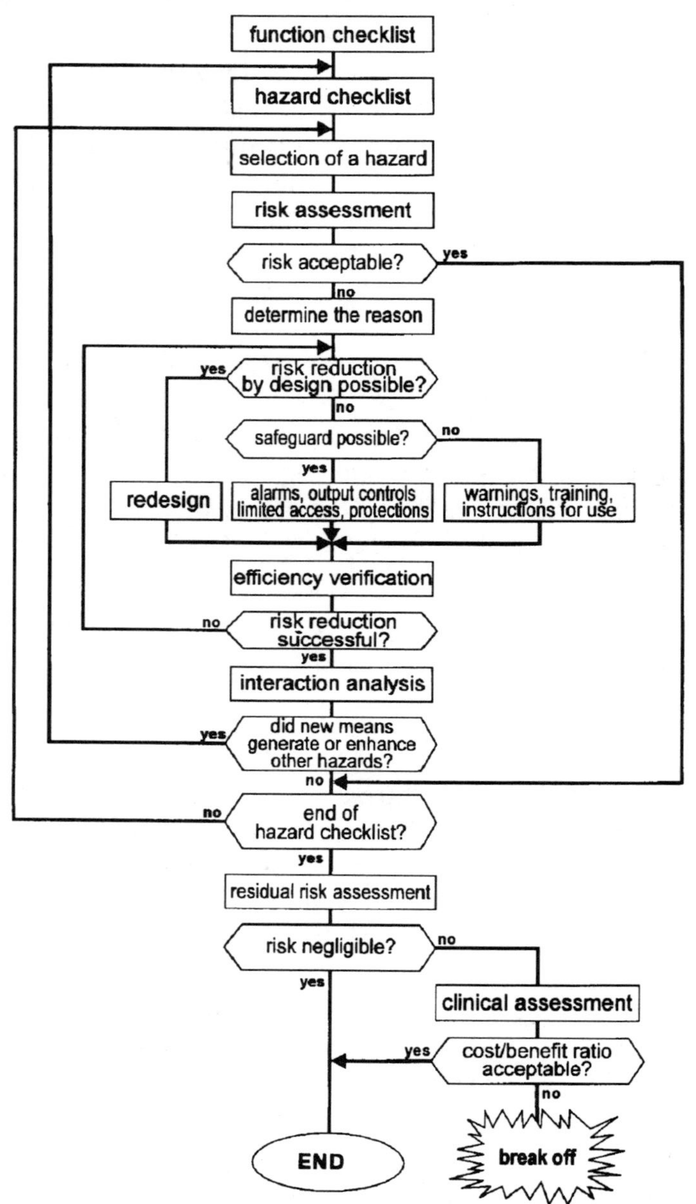

Figure 5.3. Flow diagram of the risk management process.

above 16 A might not be acceptable for common mains socket outlets. Finally, it would be necessary to look at possible warnings to see whether installation or necessary environmental conditions require additional precautions or whether for safe application special reference is made to the instructions for use.

To provide the user and the test engineer with this information, the manufacturer is obliged to put on each device a "visiting card" in the form of a permanently affixed marking. In most cases it is mounted at the rear of the device and contains the most important information, mainly in the form of numbers and symbols. To really understand the meaning, it is necessary to be acquainted with the most common symbols. Make yourself a test and try to identify the meaning of the example in Figure 5.4!

The design of the label is up to the various companies. In Figure 5.4 the first field contains the national safety labels of Austria, Germany, and Switzerland, indicating that the device has passed the full type test in these countries (or at least that the type test results of the initial body—according to certification acceptance schemes—have been accepted by the following bodies). In addition, the CE mark indicates conformity with the essential requirements (chapter 2). Because laser equipment is classified as class IIb, the conformity assessment process requires the involvement of a notified body, the identification of which is provided by the number near the CE mark.

The second field contains information on the device—the manufacturer, the type identification, the serial number, the date of production, and the electrical rated values. In the present example, the nominal current amplitude is 18 A. This means that the device

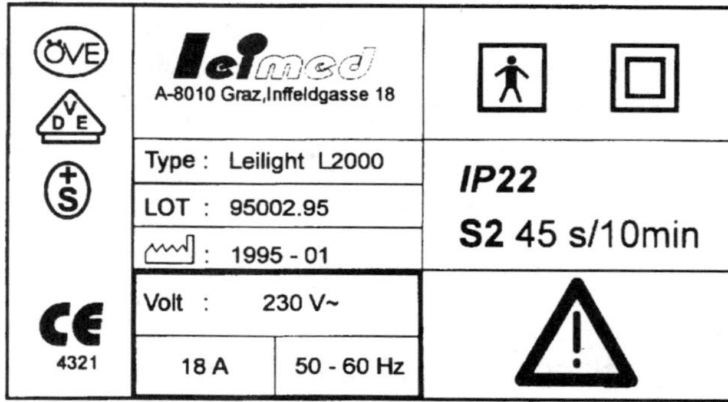

Figure 5.4. Type label of a double-insulated medical electrical device with a floating applied part; live parts are protected against touch with fingers. There is no special humidity protection; the device is for short-term use. Knowing the instructions for use is important for safe application.

must not be connected to the common mains socket outlets, which are designed for a load of 16 A only.

The third field contains safety-relevant information—the symbol for medical electrical devices with floating applied part and two concentric squares indicating double insulation (protection class II). If the device contains accessible metallic parts, it should have a means to connect a potential equalization conductor. Figures 5.5, 5.6, and 5.7 show additional markings that may be present on the label.

The designation "IP20" indicates the degree of protection against external influences (Immission Protection). The first figure characterizes protection against penetration of mechanical parts; in this case the figure

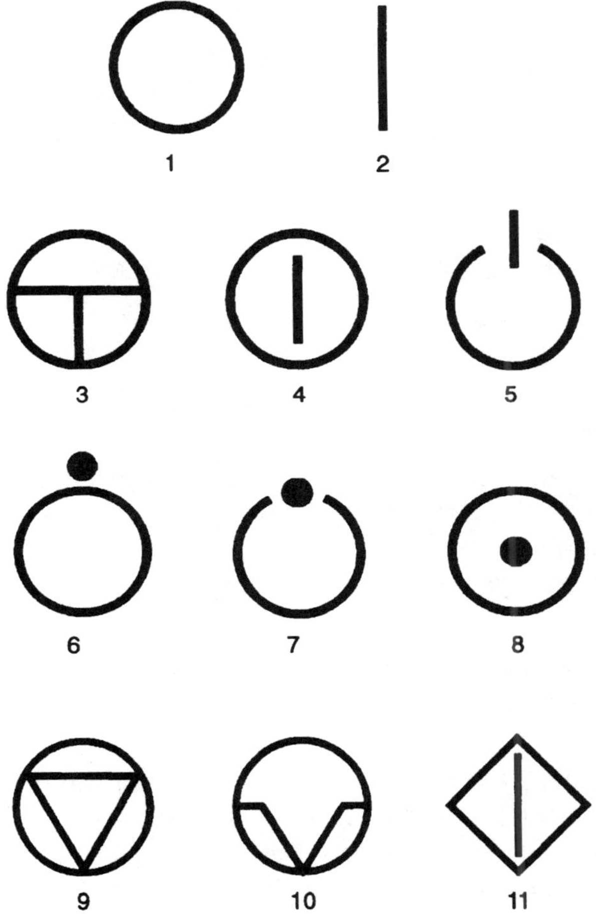

Figure 5.5. Symbols for marking switch positions: 1—Power (mains connection) on; 2—Power (mains connection) off; 3—on/off (press button); 4—on/off (touch switch); 5—device standby; 6—device part switched off; 7—device part standby; 8—device part switched on; 9—device function switched off; 10—device function standby; 11—device function switched on.

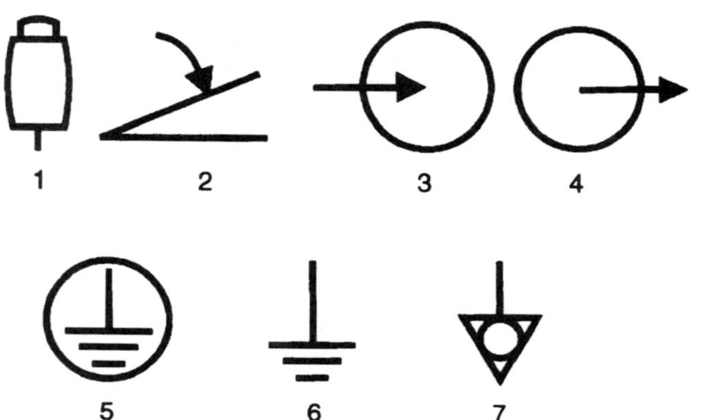

Figure 5.6. Symbols for connection points: 1—hand switch terminal; 2—foot switch terminal; 3—signal input; 4—signal output; 5—protective earth terminal; 6—(functional) earth terminal (ground); 7—equipotential terminal.

"2" indicates that life parts are protected against contacts with fingers (Table 5.1a).

Table 5.1b indicates humidity protection; the figure "0" indicates no special protection against the ingress of liquids. This means that the device may have a detachable mains cord or cooling slots, even at the top.

Medical electrical devices must be at least IP20!

The label "S2" characterizes the kind of operation; in this case it means that the device is not intended for continuous operation but is for short-term use only: it can be operated for 45 seconds, which must be followed by a break of at least 45 minutes. This duty cycle allows cooling down to starting temperature (Table

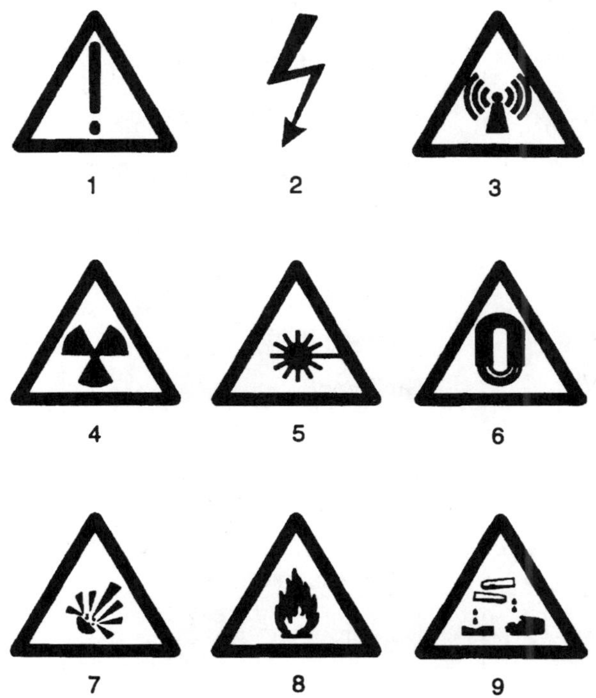

Figure 5.7. Warnings: 1—Attention, see instructions for use! 2—Attention, dangerous voltage! 3—Attention, nonionizing radiation! 4—Attention, radioactive (ionizing) radiation! 5—Attention, laser radiation! 6—Attention, high magnetic fields! 7—Attention, explosion hazard! 8—Attention, fire hazard! 9—Attention, caustic hazard!

5.2). If such labelling is not given, the device can be considered to be designed for unrestricted operation.

The warning triangle means "attention, see instructions for use" and indicates that special instructions

Abbreviation	Degree of Mechanical Protection
IP0X	No special protection
IP1X	Protected to touch with back of the hand
IP2X	Protected to touch with fingers
IP3X	Protected to touch with tools
IP4X	Protected to touch with wires
IP5X	Dust protected
IP6X	Dustproof

Table 5.1a. The Degree of Immission Protection—Mechanical

Abbreviation	Degree of Moisture Protection
IPX0	No special protection
IPX1	Drip-proof
IPX2	Rainproof
IPX3	Spray-proof
IPX4	Splash-proof
IPX5	Jet-proof
IPX6	High pressure jet-proof
IPX7	Immersion-proof
IPX8	Waterproof

Table 5.1b. The Degree of Immission Protection—Humidity

are to be followed. This warning does not have to be included in the type label but can be found on the front side (e.g., at the patient connection terminal or at critical output controls as well).

Abbreviation	Operation	Characteristic
S1	Continuous	Unlimited operation
S2	Short term	Break sufficient for cooling to initial temperature
S3	Interrupted	Break sufficient for cooling to standby temperature
Not defined	Continuous with short-term load	Break sufficient for cooling to standby temperature
Not defined	Continuous with interrupted load	Break not sufficient for cooling to standby temperature

Table 5.2. Characterization of the Intended Duration of Use

5.4 Visual Inspection

The ancient Greeks knew that we cannot see the world as it really is. If we did not continuously and automatically reduce the overwhelming amount of information that enters our eye to those small contents that are essential for survival, our brain would be hopelessly overtaxed. On the one hand, the selection of information is determined by *congenital behavior:* This is why adults recognize the typical body shape of the other sex with high priority. We all know that product promotion makes extensive use of this. On the other hand, and this is especially important with regard to safety considerations, our personal *background, experiences,* and *interests* also determine what kind of information we recognize. So someone who likes fashion tends to recognize designer clothing automatically, while car enthusiasts seldom fail to notice the various car models they encounter. Investigations show that even after we have seen the political news, we remember those items that deal with the political party we prefer.

As for safety inspections, this means that it is not sufficient just "to open eyes"! The person who does not know where to look will not be able to detect many safety deficiencies. But knowledge is not sufficient; a systematic approach and self-discipline are of similar importance. One whose attention confusedly jumps from one obvious deficiency to another, as a rule, will miss many others.

**Visual inspection requires knowledge,
a systematic approach, and self-discipline!**

In spite of the requirement to produce devices according to the technical rules, the obligation to conscientiousness, and the product liability law, which makes the manufacturer also liable for consequential damages caused by his product and which obliges him to prove his innocence (rather than to require his responsibility to be proven), the rule is that devices that have not undergone an independent safety test do not meet all the safety requirements. This is not necessarily due to the intention of the manufacturer to reduce costs, but is obviously caused by the fact that design is still based primarily on the realization of the intended function, and that awareness of safety requirements or the knowledge of safety standards is given a minor priority. **From this it follows that for newly bought devices it is absolutely vital to make a careful visual inspection, preferably before the invoice has been processed for payment!**

Careful visual inspection of (untested) new devices prevents problems later!

The goal of visual inspection, naturally, is dependent on motivation. There are three cases to be differentiated:

1. **Routine** periodic visual **inspection by the user** is made at short intervals (e.g., daily or weekly), to assure the proper condition and function of a device. It never can be excluded that the device was damaged because it was dropped, that while it was being cleaned or used for emergency treatment liquid spilled onto it, that the insulation of the mains cord was damaged, or that the device was soiled. All of these things can easily be detected by an external visual inspection. If this leads to doubts about whether there are some problems with the device, a technician should be called for internal visual inspection and measurement of safety parameters.

2. **Periodic inspections** of devices already in use are made by a clinical engineer at intervals of six months to three years. They start with an external visual inspection, which is followed by routine measurement of safety-relevant parameters, such as protective earth resistance and leakage currents. If a device has been previously checked, the technician can assume that the basic design of the device has already been accepted. (If not, he proceeds with an internal visual inspection.) In this case his attention concentrates on the presence of possible use- or age-related

safety problems. If the external visual inspection gives some indication that inside the device there are some safety-relevant changes, internal visual inspection must be performed.

3. An **initial inspection** should be performed prior to the first use of a device. It requires special attention to the external features as well as the internal ones, concentrating especially on design details, air clearances, creepage distances, and the checkpoints that are discussed below on external and internal visual inspection. All deficiencies that are not detected at this time increase risk and may cause problems later.

5.4.1 External Visual Inspection

At the beginning of each visual inspection, it is necessary to identify the device as an *individual,* that is, not only to check for the type but also for the serial number! This is especially necessary if, as in hospitals, other devices of the same type are used. But even if this is not the case, the device could have been exchanged without your knowledge because of complaints, could have been left as a substitute during repair of the initial one, and so on.

After inspection of the **type label,** and the identification of the protection class and the electrical installation requirements, the particular inspection can start. So as not to miss anything, it is important to proceed each time in the same way (Figure 5.8).

First of all we concentrate on the **enclosure:** If plastic is used, carefully look at mechanical weak points, such as cooling grids and cooling slots. If metal covers

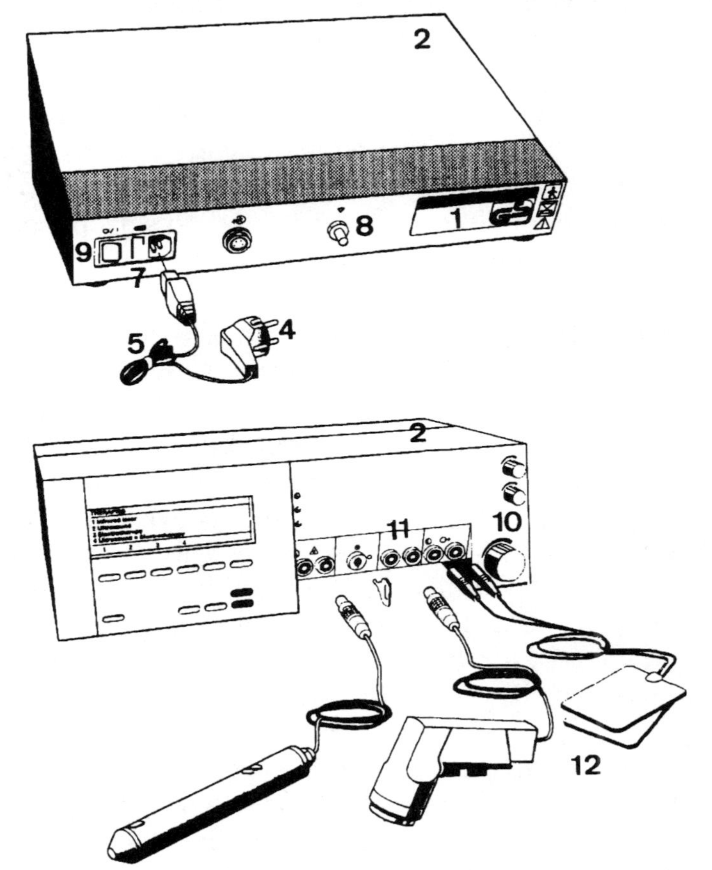

Figure 5.8. Checkpoints for external visual inspection: 1—device identification; 2—enclosure; 3—stability; 4—mains plug; 5—mains cord; 6—mains entrance point; 7—fuses; 8—potential equalization terminal; 9—mains switch; 10—operating elements; 11—(patient) terminals; 12—accessories.

are used, pay attention to deformations or dents. Signs of damage, deformation, thermally caused changes of color, extensive dust, or the occlusion of filters need increased attention. If they are detected, an internal visual inspection is imperative to check whether there are safety-relevant changes.

Protection against electric shock is inadequate if live parts (such as soldering points or even basic insulated wires) can be touched through openings or *even after the removal of any cover,* provided this is possible without using a tool.

**Everything that is accessible without tools
is considered to be touchable!**

Devices should not become **unstable** in any position of normal use. Problems may arise if devices are small and high (e.g., laboratory equipment), with the mains cord entrance point near the top, or if there are different ways to incline the device (e.g., infrared radiation devices), if there are extension arms (e.g., dental X-ray units), or if the device can carry an additional load (e.g., patient lifts, motor-driven patient chairs).

The next checkpoints are the **mains connection means:** The mains **cord** and the mains **plug** are the parts with the highest damage probability. Visual inspection includes the necessity of opening the mains plug (if not molded on) and checking for proper clamping, the adequate length of the protective earth conductor, and verifying that the cord is relieved of strain. Then the mains cord is inspected along its whole length to assure that its insulation is free of any damage.

At the device **entrance point** the cord must be protected against excessive bending (e.g., by an insulating cord guard of sufficient length, or by adequate shape of the inlet zone, like a trumpetlike opening; a metal spiral, which had formerly been used for electric irons, is no longer allowed). Absence of bending protection can be accepted at permanently installed devices only.

Devices must have cable anchorages that **relieve** conductors **from strain and twisting.** It must not be possible to pull the mains cord out or to push it into the device (relieving strain by making a knot in the cable is not acceptable!).

Fuses that are accessible from the outside frequently are weak points of protection. Fuse holders must be constructed so that it is not possible to touch live contacts, either directly with the sole finger or during exchange of the fuse. (There are specially protected fuse holders available that are nearly twice as deep as the nonprotected ones.)

The **number** of necessary mains fuses depends on the protection class of the device: For double-insulated devices in general, a single fuse is sufficient, whereas protectively earthed devices need fuses in every active mains conductor. Thus, general class I devices should be provided with at least two fuses. If, on external inspection, no fuse at all or an insufficient number of fuses can be found, the device might still meet the requirements; it is acceptable for some or even all mains fuses to be placed inside the device. If there are doubts, this should be clarified by internal inspection. It should also be routine to include a check as to whether the rated values of the used fuses correspond with the nominal values (which must be marked near the fuse holder!). It is not uncommon that in cases of blown fuses the technician does not have an adequate spare fuse available and uses another one provisionally, which is often not replaced with a correct one later. Therefore, it is important that there be someone in the safety system who regularly checks fuses in use for appropriate values.

After the fuses, the last mains part that can be inspected from the outside is **the mains switch.** If no mains switch is present, it is allowed that devices have another means for complete separation from mains. Mains plugs are accepted for this purpose as well. However, if present, mains switches must meet all relevant requirements: They must interrupt each mains conductor, and the clearance (from 50 V to 400 V) must be at least 3 mm. It is not uncommon to find "microswitches" with reduced clearances for switching mains voltage: If there are doubts, internal visual inspection will reveal that such (insufficient) switches are marked with a "μ".

In contrast to household devices, mains switches must not be incorporated in a power supply cord or any external flexible lead. It is up to the manufacturer to decide where the mains switch is mounted, but the switching positions must be clearly marked. To prevent human error, the "on" position must be to the right or upward. If an indicator lamp is used, it must be green.

Red lamps are allowed for danger indication only!

Up to now we have concentrated on protective aspects. We now move on to functional items. **Operating elements** must be reliably fixed on the shaft. They must be checked to verify that the reading is in accord with the indicated minimum and maximum positions.

All **connections** (plugs and sockets) must prevent hazardous interchanges. This applies especially to plugs for patient circuit leads. Here is an example of a Murphy's law accident. When a mother visited her child, the electrocardiogram cables were detached from a device to allow the child to move. At the end of the visit, the mother wanted to reconnect the cables. So she looked at the banana plugs and searched for the possible connection points. Detecting the red-colored emergency power socket outlet above the bed, she believed she had found the right connection and plugged in the cables. This resulted in a fatal electric shock to her child. To prevent similar accidents (and to prevent accidental grounding of a patient's circuit as well), banana plugs that fit into mains socket outlets must not be used, and, of course, devices must not have related sockets for patient circuits.

An important and final part of the external visual inspection is the **function test.** It is important to emphasize that safety checks should be restricted deliberately to safety-relevant functions. The check of performance and accuracy or calibration is and should remain the responsibility of the user, who must check for this much more frequently than is common for safety inspections. It could be a fateful misunderstanding if the user believes that this is no longer required because periodic safety checks cover this aspect. The function test, therefore, is primarily intended to check whether the technical conditions for safety-relevant functions, such as alarms or warning lights, are working. However, if the alarm settings must be changed for testing, they must either be put in the initial position or the device must be clearly marked as having altered alarm limits.

If the external visual inspection is made by a technician, it must be accompanied by the **measurement** of safety-relevant parameters, such as protective earth resistance or leakage currents. Depending on the device, of course, *safety-relevant* output parameters must also be checked (e.g., the energy of the defibrillator impulse, the infusion rate of an infusion pump, the output power of a high frequency surgical device, and the light intensity of therapeutic laser equipment).

5.4.2 Internal Visual Inspection

While an external visual inspection can and should be made by the user, the inspection of the interior of a device is restricted to competent persons who are trained and are aware of the possible hazards that can result if the device's protective enclosure is removed.

First of all, it must be determined whether it is possible to open a device at all. In principle, only the new editions of standards -IEC 601-1/1988 or EN 60601-1/1990 allow for the design of fail-safe devices that do not require repair, but in case of a failure are replaced by a new one. In these cases it is permitted to seal the devices permanently and prevent access to the interior. However, if maintenance is intended that requires the opening of the device, this must be possible without causing any damage. This applies as well if, during the lifetime of a device, internal inspections are necessary to assure safety.

The visual inspection of the interior of a device, in particular, requires a systematic approach (Figure 5.9). It is recommended to start with an inspection of the wiring of all mains parts from the entrance point of the mains cable to the separation from the applied part; then to inspect the insulation of accessible parts, the applied part, and the used electronic components; and, finally, to look for signs of excessive heating or mechanical damage. Increased attention is necessary

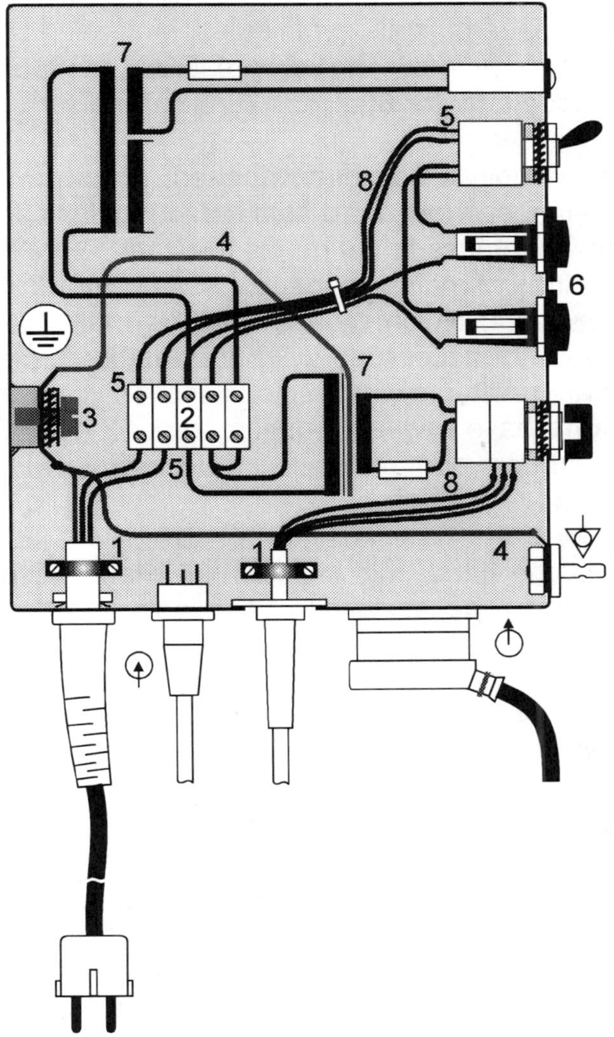

Figure 5.9. Checkpoints for internal visual inspection: 1—mains cable entrance; 2—mains terminal; 3—protective earth terminal; 4—protective earth connections; 5—internal wiring; 6—fuses; 7—transformer; 8—separation (clearance, creepage distance); 9—components; 10—signs of overheating; 11—mechanical fixation; 12—signs of abrasion.

if additional risk factors are combined with the intended use (e.g., spilling of liquids, increased concentrations of oxygen, or the presence of flammable gases [see chapter 6]).

Once the device has been opened, the **strain relief** can be inspected in more detail at the mains cable entrance. Then pass to the mains terminal. There are different kinds of mains connections: **Z connections** are not rewirable, which means that the mains terminal device is not accessible without damage; **Y connections** are rewirable with a special tool only; and **X connections** have rewirable mains cords. X connections are most common and must be accessible with common tools.

On the one hand, this implies that **mains terminals** must not be accessible without tools. On the other hand, it follows that medical equipment with a mains cable does require a mains terminal device. Connection with internal wiring only, by freely moving wire-to-wire soldering, does not meet the requirement. If the connection is made by clamping, it should be designed such that the conductor may not be damaged and cannot slip out when clamping screws are tightened. This can be assured by using a terminal with metal tongues between the screws and the wires. Mains terminal devices must be insulated or positioned such that an accidentally escaping wire (of 8 mm length) neither reduces safety-relevant insulation nor comes into contact with other live parts. In many cases this requirement makes it necessary to have an insulating layer beneath the mounting block. It is explicitly forbidden to clamp soldered wires with screws! The reason for this is the low melting point of solder, which is responsible for deformation at the contact area at comparable low temperatures and leads to worsening of the contact, which then increases heating. Because of this positive feedback, the reliability of such contacts is significantly decreased. Instead of soldering stranded wires, use end sleeves!

Clamped wires must not be soldered!

Reliability of the **connection with the ground** is especially important for protectively earthed devices. Therefore, some rules should be observed: Clamp connections must be protected against accidental loosening (e.g., by lock washers). The positioning of terminal points and/or the length of the protective earth conductor must assure that in case of mechanical strain the protective earth connection fails last. The connection should have a low resistance (which, between accessible metal parts and the mains plug, must not exceed **0.2 Ω**). Although the protective earth resistance can be checked only by measurement, visual inspection is helpful: Attention should be paid to whether the cross section of the protective earth wire, at least up to the fuses, is not lower than those of the mains conductors. It is recommended to have a central earth terminal. It is alarming if the protective earth connection is performed via electronic circuit boards. Reductions of cross sections must be considered very critically; printed circuits rarely exhibit the necessary cross-sectional areas for protective earth interconnections.

The single-fault condition must be assumed at each **connection point** of a wire, irrespective of whether it is in the mains or a secondary part! Therefore, at any terminal point the consequences of a break or a loosening of the wire must be considered. If the loosened wire could come into contact with accessible metal parts or safety-relevant circuits, the conductor must be mechanically secured by independent means. In most cases it is sufficient to use a cable binder to fix two or more wires together mechanically (because the loosening of more than one conductor at the same time is not considered to be a single fault). Another solution would be fixation by shrink-down tubes or bending solid wires around the fixation hole before soldering.

The loosening of a wire at the connection point must always be considered!

From the mains terminal device follow the wiring to the **mains fuses.** Unlike household devices, medical electrical devices must be provided with overcurrent protection means (fuses): Double-insulated devices need at least *one* fuse; protectively earthed devices need a fuse in every active mains conductor (that means at least *two*). Double-insulated devices now are allowed to have an earth connection, but only for functional reasons (e.g., for shielding) rather than for safety. In this case, with regard to overcurrent protection, these devices must be treated like protectively earthed devices that require more than one fuse.

The most important component for safety is the **mains transformer.** Its task is not only to transform the mains voltage into the several voltage levels needed by the device but also to provide separation between the secondary circuits and the mains. This can be achieved in different ways: by using double chamber coil frames with separated coils for primary and secondary windings, or by a common coil frame where both coils are wound one over the other and are separated by insulating layers.

Safety deficiencies in the design of transformers are most common. The reason is that it is not sufficient to have thick insulation; one must also make sure that any pathway through which electrical currents could flow to the secondary winding or to the earthed iron transformer core across cracks and rents or along surfaces has sufficient length. For double insulation (between primary and secondary winding), the necessary creepage distance is 8 mm; for basic insulation (to the earthed core) it is 4 mm. The insulating varnish of the winding allows a reduction of the distances by 1 mm. Weak points with creepage distances too small are commonly found across the separating wall of double chamber coil frames and at their corners at the iron core (Figure 5.10). Frequently found, but difficult to detect by visual inspection, are creepage distance insufficiencies at single chamber windings. They can be found at the separating layers if they are ending up with the end of the coil instead of being extended and bent upward to increase creepage distances.

The next step of inspection is to follow the **internal wiring** and to pay attention to whether the double insulation between mains and secondary circuits is provided throughout all pathways. This means that conductors, even with basic insulation, are not allowed to contact bare (soldering) points of double-insulated circuits. A force (of 2 N) may be applied to bring a cable into the most unfavorable position and verify that such contact still does not occur. Insulating tubes must be applied such that either they cannot move or that even after shifting the insulation is still provided. However, these checks must be done carefully and restricted to those cases that cannot be decided otherwise. It can be observed that even experienced persons tend to make this kind of test too

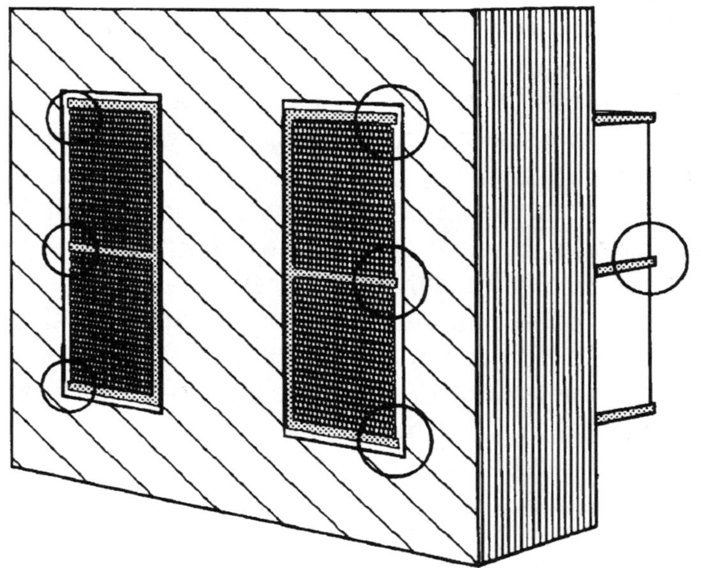

Figure 5.10. Safety-relevant (commonly weak) points at a transformer.

rigidly. **It must be assured that the device is not tested to death and that it is not made worse than before!**

If wires of two circuits with different voltages (e.g., the mains voltage, the logic voltage level, the teletube voltage, or the high voltage for laser tubes) touch each other, the insulation of a conductor must be at least electrically equivalent to the others, otherwise the conductor must be regarded as bare with the insulation thickness as air clearance. Nonequivalent conductors must be positioned such that touching of critical conductors is prevented or they must be surrounded by an additional insulation.

Conductors with insufficient insulation
are considered to be bare!

Visual inspection of the internal wiring must not only concentrate on electrical aspects, but should include two further aspects as well. On the one hand, there are the **mechanical influences.** It must be determined whether there is a risk of friction or squeezing. Critical points are feed-throughs or adjacent moving parts, such as ventilator wings, motors, or swinging arms. On the other hand, the device must be checked for possible **overheating.** PVC insulation is not allowed to be exposed to temperatures over 75°C, because it could become stiff and rent (at movable cables, such as mains cords, temperatures must not exceed 60°C). A danger of overheating can arise at the mains transformer, power resistances, output amplifiers, infrared bulbs, and, of course, near dedicated heating elements.

Color coding of internal wiring is unrestricted, with one exception: Ground connectors, irrespective of whether they are intended for protection, potential equilibration, shielding, or functional aspects, must be yellow/green (with one color part not being less than 30 percent) along the *whole length* of the conductor! If there are places where this cannot be realized (e.g., at flexible bare potential equilibration conductors in large equipment such as X-ray computer tomographs), or if several leads of a multiple lead cable are used together to achieve a sufficient cross section, it is allowed to durably mark such components yellow/green at both ends only. To surround the conductor ends with a friction tape cannot be considered durable marking if loosening is not prevented by additional means.

After having inspected the internal wiring, progress to the bare live parts and check **air clearances** and **creepage distances.** Air is allowed to be used for insulation provided that the safety distances are assured for the whole lifetime of the device, even if a force is applied to the parts that must be separated. The air clearance is measured as the shortest distance between the parts that must be insulated from each other. The necessary length depends on the acting voltage. For basic insulation the absolute minimum is 0.8 mm; for double insulation the value must be doubled (Table 5.3). For mains voltage (230 V), air clearance should not be lower than 2.5 mm (5 mm for double insulation). Increased attention is necessary if printed circuits are extended up to the edge of an electronic board. Problems commonly may arise concerning distances from protectively earthed parts to the soldering side of a print board, to bare (deformable!) soldering tags, or to bare connection wires (e.g., from resistances).

The absolute minimum air clearance is 0.8 mm!

Since leakage currents can flow even across insulation, it must be considered that they can flow along surfaces or cracks and rents, especially if these are soiled. It is, therefore, required that the **creepage distance** along the surface between bare conductors (or across rents) must not be below the given limits. Bare conductors are not uncommon within devices: They may not only be soldering tags, soldering points, or bare connection wires of components—most of all they may be conductors of printed circuits. Varnish generally is not considered insulation, but may be considered as soiling protection. In printed circuits this is taken into account by reducing distances in comparison with unprotected cases. Creepage distance is

		15	36	75	150	300	450	600	800	900	1200
DC Voltage (in volts)		15	36	75	150	300	450	600	800	900	1200
AC Voltage (in volts)		12	30	60	125	250	380	500	660	750	1000
Basic Insulation (between Opposite Poles)	Air Clearance (in mm)	0.4	0.5	0.7	1	1.6	2.4	3	4	4.5	6
	Creepage Distance (in mm)	0.8	1	1.3	2	3	4	5.5	7	8	11
Basic Insulation (Supplementary Insulation)	Air Clearance (in mm)	0.8	1	1.2	1.6	2.5	3.5	4.5	6	6.5	9
	Creepage Distance (in mm)	1.7	2	2.3	3	4	6	8	10.5	12	16
Double or Reinforced Insulation	Air Clearance (in mm)	1.6	2	2.4	3.2	5	7	9	12	13	18
	Creepage Distance (in mm)	3.4	4	4.6	6	8	12	16	21	24	32

Table 5.3. Air Clearance and Creepage Distances Independent of Voltage

defined as the shortest path along surfaces (or across cracks). Grooves of any depth are not taken into account if their width is smaller than 1 mm (Figure 5.11). The creepage distances also depend on the voltage to be insulated. The minimum distance is 1.7 mm for basic insulation (3.4 mm for double insulation); 4 mm for mains voltage (8 mm for double insulation). In general, the creepage distance is roughly twice the necessary air clearance.

**Creepage distances are roughly
twice the air clearance.**

Internal visual inspection must include **components** as well. Their nominal values (e.g., voltage or current), must at least conform to the rated values of the device. Mains power switches and mains transformers commonly do not meet this requirement, either because American versions without modifications are also used for the European market or because they are not designed for the rated current of the device. Other components, such as electrolytic capacitors, may have indicated temperatures that are not adequate for the enhanced temperatures that are common near power resistors, cooling plates, or transformers.

Finally, pay attention to general **mechanical aspects.** Unsupported joints between wiring and components are weak points that have a high probability of loosening. They are not indicators of safe design and should be avoided. Electronic boards should be mounted at several points so that they can withstand vibration.

5.5 Corrective Measures

In practice, it is not self-evident that the requirements in regard to creepage distances and air clearances are

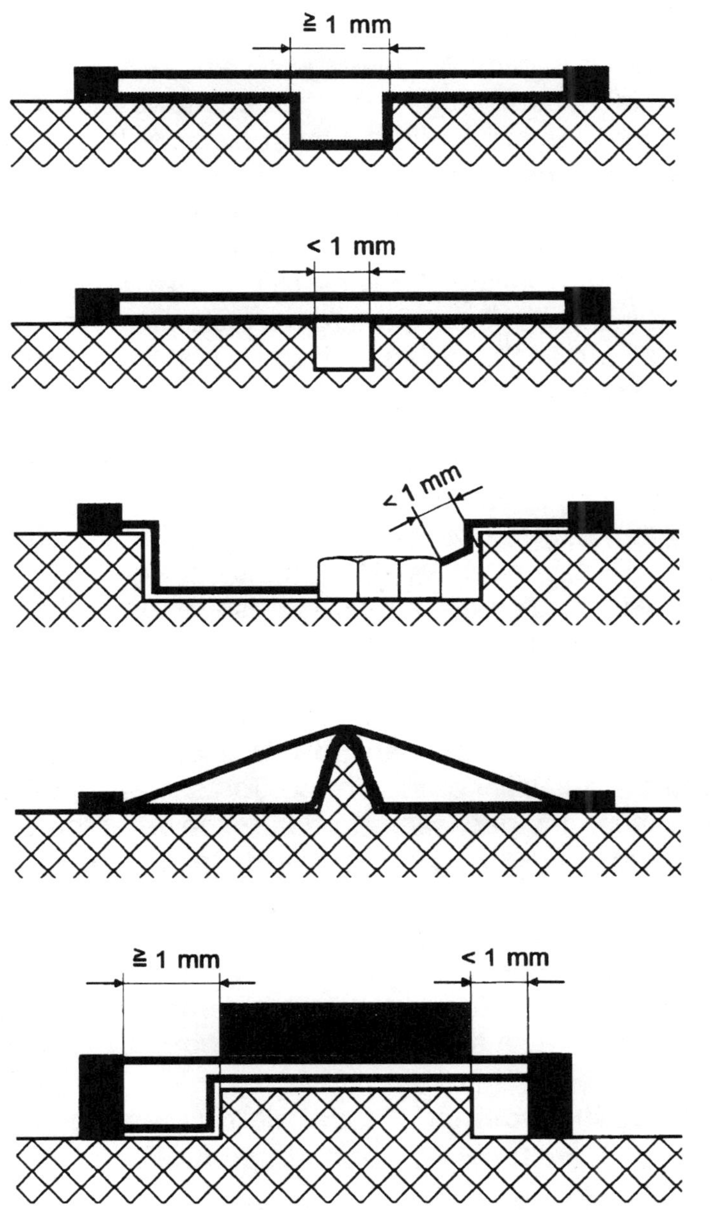

Figure 5.11. Measurement of air clearances and creepage distances.

fulfilled. However, while air clearances that are too small can be corrected by the use of additional insulation, the correction of creepage distances that are too small is not as easy. Experience shows that most shortcomings are found at electronic boards between mains and secondary conductors, at connector sockets, or near (grounded) mounting screws. Printed (metallic) markings may pose unintended difficulties. As they are electrically conducting, they may short-circuit initially sufficient clearance distances. Once difficulties are encountered, it must be clarified how they can be overcome.

At **entrance checks** the situation would be more comfortable for the tester: He could define the problem and then threaten the company by making the settlement of the bill dependent on an adequate correction. However, with equipment already in use, one must solve the problem on his own.

First of all, the safety relevance of the deficient creepage distance must be clarified. It is clear that it may reduce the reliability of the device. To assess the safety relevance, it is necessary to determine what the consequences would be if the creepage distance were short-circuited. It must be emphasized, that, because of the distance reduction, this must **not** be considered a single-fault condition! This means that even leakage currents (earth, enclosure, and patient leakage currents) must meet the limit values for *normal* condition!

A short circuit of a deficient creepage distance is not a single fault!

Deficient creepage distances should be avoided. However, in a concession to reality, specific reductions of creepage distances can be tolerated under the following constraints:

- In the *mains part* **between opposite polarity** if this occurs *beyond the fuses.* In this case a short circuit of these creepage distances would be harmless and would only cause blown fuses.

- If the creepage distance provides **basic insulation** (e.g., between the applied part and the enclosure), and if short circuiting does not increase the enclosure leakage current beyond the limits for *normal* conditions.

If these additional conditions are fulfilled, no other measures are necessary. But even in more critical cases, deficient creepage distances should not be accepted as an unavoidable source of problems. A redesign with an improved layout of the electronic board would be the best, albeit expensive, solution. There are several alternatives here as well:

- Frequent problems can be found at **the mains cord terminal block** (which is located before the fuses!). Recall that an 8 mm long free wire of a stranded conductor must not come into contact with the protectively earthed enclosure. In most cases the use of an additional insulation foil beneath the terminal might be sufficient, if it extends beyond it by sufficient length.

- If a free wire is able to contact the neighbouring conductor, the use of a longer terminal block with spare terminals between the clamped conductors might be sufficient. If not, insulating plates can be mounted between the terminal points.

- At electronic boards deficient creepage distances can be corrected in different ways:

  — The easiest, although unattractive, solution is to cover the critical distances with an adhesive, nonthermoplastic casting compound (varnishing is not sufficient).

  — Frequently, creepage distances are too small only at limited critical sites, commonly where edges of conductors approach another circuit too closely. In such cases it might be sufficient to round the extending edge.

  — If the creepage distance is not smaller than the necessary air clearance, another solution is to mill a groove not less than 1 mm wide into the printing board. By doing this, the distance can be considered as air clearance that requires only about half the necessary creepage length. Of course, this must not impair the mechanical properties of the board to a safety-relevant extent.

  — If the creepage distance is too small along a longer pathway, a possible solution is to interrupt this pathway along a sufficient length and to replace it by an external wire. However, in this case it must be determined what happens if this wire is loosened at the soldering points (single-fault condition) and whether requirements for double insulation are fulfilled even if the wire is shifted as far as possible.

5.6 Medical Systems

Last but not least, progress in medicine, especially in medical technology, also reflects development in other technical fields. It has not only opened new possibilities (e.g., to make cross-sectional X-ray images of the brain by computer tomography), but has also led to the application of complex combinations of different devices (for instance, ultrasound scanners, which may consist of a scanner, computer, monitor, video recorder, thermoprinter, and a camera). Modern technology even involves the installation of extended systems, such as magnetic resonance imagers, which may have components in different, even nonmedically used, rooms. It is typical that such systems may consist of components that initially were designed and tested for an intended use other than a medical application. The situation is complicated by the fact that components may also be installed in nonmedically used rooms with a power supply system that may only meet less stringent requirements in regard to protective earth resistance, SELV, or power supply reliability (see chapter 7).

Even if all devices meet the requirements for their (main) intended use, it must be considered whether and under what conditions they may be incorporated within a complex system for medical application. In fact, medical **systems** may cause additional risks for the following reasons:

- Because of interconnections, leakage currents may be critically enhanced if particular standards for some of the components permit higher values than are permitted for medical devices.

- If several components are supplied by a common mains cord, the interruption of the protective earth conductor may lead to a critically enhanced enclosure leakage current.

- Different components of the system may be connected to different electrical circuits, even in different rooms. This could have two consequences: On the one hand, different protective earth resistors and earth leakage currents may lead to significant potential differences between parts of the system. On the other hand, initially separated protective earth conductors may be connected to loops that, like antennas, might pick up electromagnetic noise, which can increase electromagnetic interference.

- Special attention is paid to the separation between mains voltage and applied parts for medical electrical devices. Because of less stringent requirements for nonmedical devices, the probability of introducing critical voltages to the patient may be enhanced.

- Extended signal connections to other devices (e.g., from the intensive care unit to the central monitoring facilities), may also act like antennas and pick up electromagnetic noise, which, in turn, may affect the devices.

- Signal voltages of grounded circuits, even at safe levels, may lead to excessive patient leakage currents. (For example, under a single-fault condition, 242 V at the signal input are allowed to enhance the patient leakage current up to 5 mA. Therefore, (grounded) voltages of not more than 4.8 V may cause the patient leakage current to exceed the limit for a normal condition of 0.1 mA.)

According to standard EN 60601-1-1, these problems can be solved in different ways:

- The hazard potential is different in different parts of a medically used room, with the area surrounding the patient as the most critical zone. Therefore, it has been determined that all equipment that is used within the **patient environment** (see Figure 4.9) must meet the requirements for medical electrical devices, at least in regard to leakage currents. As indicated in Figure 4.9, the patient environment is defined as the zone within a distance of 1.5 m from the intended position of the patient. If devices do not fulfill this condition, it can be met by using an insulating transformer that provides a floating power supply (see chapter 3). Another possibility is to place those devices outside the critical zone.

- To avoid any possible danger due to grounded signal voltages, the connection with nonmedical devices requires an additional potential separation. If this is not already incorporated within the device, external separation means, such as optical couplings, should be provided as close to the medical device as possible.

- To avoid the risk of excessive enhancement of the enclosure leakage current due to the interruption of the common protective earth conductor, an additional (external) protective earth conductor should be used as a redundant safety precaution.

It can be concluded that electromedical devices can be used without further safety precautions, even in combination with each other. However, if the system contains at least one nonmedical device, additional precautions may be necessary, such as a further protective earth connection, the use of an insulating transformer, or additional means for separation within the signal lines (Figure 5.12).

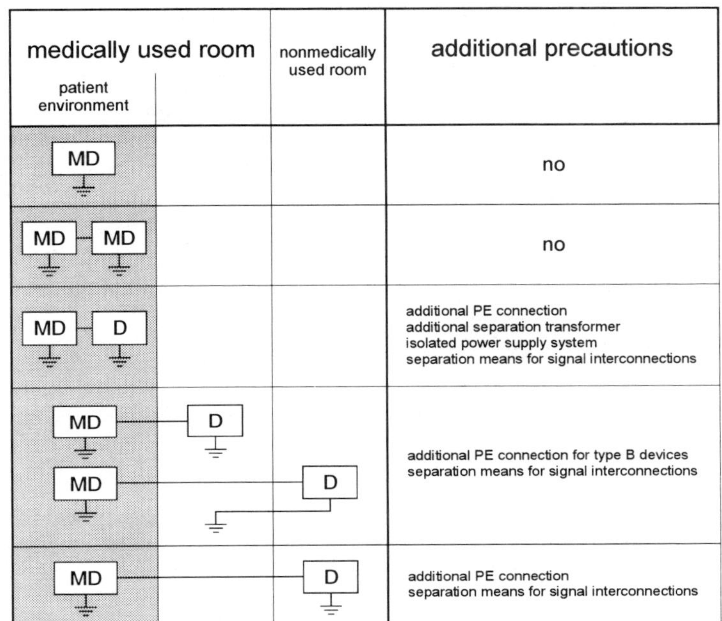

Figure 5.12. Additional safety precautions for medical systems.

6 Dangerous Cofactors

Familiarity with situations in daily life makes daily routine much easier: It enables us to do things without thinking about them again and again. For instance, when walking, we rely on adhesive friction being large enough to enable us to put our feet on the ground safely. The same situation, however, could demand quite a different behaviour if oil has been spilled or if there is an unexpected frost. Similarly, smokers assume that ashes falling from their cigarette will not cause any harm. In most cases, this is true. However, if the oxygen content of the air or the smoker's clothing is increased, as it is, for instance, after having been within an oxygen tent, the same inconspicuous ignition source can be sufficient to lead to a dangerous fire on the clothing.

In a medical environment additional risk factors are not rare. They might be combined with the use of liquids, oxygen, or flammable gases; or with the presence of pathogenic germs. In each case they require increased attention by medical personnel and specific precautions in the construction of medical devices.

6.1 The Use of Liquids

Even humid air can be a risk factor: It might impair inadequate electrical insulation. This is why medical electrical equipment is not allowed to contain hygroscopic electrical insulation. Even after a 48-hour exposure to 98 percent humid air, devices must fulfill all requirements.

In combination with medical electrical devices, liquids constitute a particular danger: It is not surprising that in the home the most severe accidents with electricity occur in bathrooms. The reason is that most liquids, even water, have a fairly good electrical conductivity. Therefore, if introduced into a device, liquids can impair electrical insulation and even short-circuit creepage distances and air clearances. Larger amounts can become electric pathways to live parts in the interior and can make dangerous voltages accessible and protective means ineffective. Aggressive liquids, such as battery acids, can also cause chemical hazards.

If the intended use of a device may require handling with liquids (e.g., infusion pumps, nerve and muscle stimulators), unintended spillage of liquids must be taken into account. This requires constructive precautions to prevent liquids, even under single-fault conditions, from wetting electrical insulation and causing hazards. In regard to constructive precautions, three cases must be differentiated:

1. Devices that **already contain liquids,** such as blood gas analyzers, must be protected from dangerous moistening in the position of normal use. For movable devices this must be assured even at an inclination of 15 degrees. For refillable containers, spilling up to 15 percent of the volume must not affect safety. Points of increased risk for the leakage of liquids are joints and branches, tube connections, and sealings. If possible, liquid-containing parts should be positioned below

electric parts to prevent those parts from contact with liquids even in single-fault conditions. Liquid-containing parts under pressure, such as water tubes in medical supply units, must be checked by the manufacturer for their tightness by overpressure tests.

2. If, during the intended use of a device, **handling with liquids** can be expected (e.g., for wetting sponge electrodes for nerve or muscle stimulation), the design must allow for accidental spilling. (This can be tested by spillage of 0.2 ℓ water at the most unfavorable point of the device.) The enclosure of such devices, therefore, must not have openings at the top. Slits between connected parts of the enclosure must be sealed or designed such that ingressing liquid cannot pose any harm. It goes without saying that parts that will contact the patient must be disinfectable and able to withstand the expected moistening.

Frequent complaints are caused by the inadequate design of cooling slots that are bent toward the interior, by mains couplings, or by mains switches. An example of insufficient protection against the ingress of liquid was found in an emergency defibrillator set. The manufacturer had been aware that the device might be used in open air, even under bad weather conditions, and had included the electronics within a part of an insulating case, the second part of which was dedicated to housing the stimulating electrodes. The electric part was covered by an insulating hood that, for maintenance reasons, was not sealed at all. It was not taken into account that although liquid could flow down from the hood, it would collect within the electrode's compartment, from where it might have enough time to enter the electronics and cause dangerous breakdowns.

3. Devices with **increased protection** against the ingress of liquids must be marked by the "IP" code (see Table 5.1b) and, of course, must fulfill the adequate requirements. Special attention must be paid to foot switches. Because they may remain on the floor even during room cleaning, they may be exposed to larger amounts of liquids. Therefore, they are required to be at least drip-proof (IPX1). If intended for use in an operation theatre, foot switches must be watertight (IPX6).

6.2 Pathogenic Germs

Germs (microorganisms) are everywhere. They can be found in the air (urban air contains up to 2,000 germs/m^3), in water (drinking water contains 10–10,000 germs/ℓ), and even on the skin or inside the body. In fact, even in a healthy condition we are germ emitters in daily life. On the skin, germs act as "garbage grinders" and are responsible for body odor; they protect us from non-resident microorganisms and play an important role in our digestion. By the touch of a single finger, we can transfer 20–100 germs/cm^2. If we sneeze, we propel from tens of thousands up to millions of germs into the air. Depending on our activity, we release 6–1,800 million particles, with approximately 1 in 1000 being germs.

Germs are everywhere!

This is why sophisticated ventilation is necessary in operation theatres to keep a high hygienic level and to ensure low germ concentration in spite of the presence of people. To ensure a germ concentration as low as 10 germs/m^3, as is required for heart transplantation, it would be necessary to replace the whole air volume of the operation theatre by adequately filtered fresh air up to 60 times per hour!

Under favorable conditions (e.g., at temperatures between 20°C and 50°C, and especially in the presence of nutritive substances), germ proliferation increases exponentially. Therefore, all liquid residues must be assumed to contain excessive numbers of germs!

In standing liquids germs increase like an avalanche!

For a healthy person, microorganisms at common concentrations are not hazardous. Patients, however, can be overstrained by excessive germ concentrations. On the other hand, patients, especially those suffering from infectious diseases, are dangerous germ sources and can cause dangerous contaminations of medical devices.

There are three ways for medical devices to become dangerous germ sources.

1. **Direct contamination,** which is due to the application of applied parts to infectious patients. In addition, adjustable knobs and handles are the most likely contaminated parts. Devices whose intended use requires direct contact with blood or other body liquids, such

as suction devices, are at highest risk. A service engineer once contracted severe hepatitis because he was given a device to repair that had been delivered from an infection station without any disinfection. Therefore, service engineers and staff of the medical technical department should ask for the place of last use before starting to work on a device.

2. **Difficult disinfection,** which in many cases is due to construction deficiencies. This can be caused by design (e.g., due to rough or structured surfaces, inaccessible recesses, undercuts, or cooling slots). Another reason can be material aging, such as rubber or synthetic tubes of anaesthetic devices, ventilation devices, valve rings, or catheters of suction devices. Disinfection is also made difficult by hard-to-disassemble seals, fittings, or tubes.

3. **Germ proliferation.** Because of the exponential multiplication of omnipresent germs, each liquid remainder constitutes a potential hygienic risk that increases with time. This must not only be considered for devices that intentionally store liquids for some period (such as inhalators, nebulizers, or electrogalvanic baths), but also for devices where liquids unintentionally can remain (as in suction devices, endoscopes, or accessories such as sponge electrodes). Problems can also arise in standing water within the (warm) water supply system or within the air conditioning equipment.

Liquid residues are hygienic risk factors!

The user must be especially careful in preparing and conducting the disinfection, and must properly dry devices and accessories. The *manufacturer* must take care of the hygienic aspects of the design and the selection of materials. For instance, a foil-covered keyboard is preferred over a set of individual push buttons. In any case, however, all parts that are intended to come into contact with the patient must withstand the procedures for disinfection or sterilization that have been (and must be) specified in the instructions for use.

6.3 Oxygen

Oxygen has two quite different aspects: On the one hand, it is beneficial and of utmost importance for life; on the other hand, it is responsible for considerable danger. Burning, irrespective of whether it takes place within our body or in the external environment, can occur only if sufficient oxygen is available. The oxygen content of air is 21 percent. It is responsible for the flammability and burn behaviour of substances familiar to us. However, an increase of this figure by just a few percentage points is sufficient to cause dramatic changes both in flammability and burn behavior. In an **oxygen-enriched atmosphere** (with oxygen content of 4 percent more than normal) burns occur easier, proceed faster, and produce higher temperatures.

Additional oxygen increases the probability, speed, and temperature of burns!

With additional oxygen, burns occur **more easily** because substances can be ignited by less energy. In pure oxygen the minimum ignition energy can be reduced by as much as two magnitudes. This leads to two serious consequences: (1) Common uncritical ignition sources, such as cigarette ashes or an electrostatic spark discharge, can become dangerous. (2) Things that ordinarily do not ignite suddenly burn intensely. Cotton clothing flashes at an oxygen content of only 28 percent. In device technology all organic substances, including most kinds of electrical insulation, are considered to be flammable, and oxygen enrichment (e.g., by leakage of tube connections), can contribute to insulation burns.

**In an oxygen-enriched atmosphere
PVC insulation is easily flammable!**

Fat, including face creams, lipsticks, or fat residues from foods can become dangerous in an oxygen-enriched atmosphere. This leads to the following recommendations:

**Refrain from smoking in an oxygen-
enriched atmosphere!**

Keep fat away from oxygen!

**Take care to allow sufficient ventilation
of oxygen-enriched clothes
(more than 1 hour, at a minimum)!**

With additional oxygen, burns proceed **faster** and, therefore, are more dangerous. For instance, in a 38 percent oxygen-enriched atmosphere, the burn speed of cotton clothing is increased eightfold. This is why a nurse could not be rescued when she smoked a cigarette after working with a patient in an oxygen tent. Cigarette ashes had set her clothes on fire, burning her skin before the fire could be extinguished.

In the oxygen stream of a pressure bottle, greased fittings can be ignited with an explosion-like burning of the fat. This can lead to damage of the gas bottle and to considerable consequent damage.

In an oxygen-enriched atmosphere the **burn temperature** is considerably **increased** (e.g., the temperature of cigarette ashes increases from 600°C up to 900°C).

These facts show that oxygen, although not burnable itself, significantly enhances the burn hazard. When people lack relevant experience, this risk is often underestimated. Therefore, it must be learned, hopefully without an accident, that dealing with oxygen requires special risk awareness. An oxygen-enriched atmosphere must not be produced carelessly. Oxygen must not needlessly be used instead of compressed air to operate pneumatic devices. Oxygen must not be used simply to improve the air quality.

**Do not needlessly use oxygen
instead of compressed air!**

It goes without saying that all oxygen-containing devices, such as anaesthetic machines, lung ventilators, and incubators, require additional safety precautions:

- Electrical parts must be separated from regions where, even under single-fault conditions, an oxygen-enriched atmosphere can develop (e.g., by placement or capsulation). They must be prevented from being exposed to increased oxygen concentrations of more than 4 percent above normal. Oxygen is heavier than air, and leakage accumulates at the bottom of a device. Oxygen-containing parts should be positioned below electrical parts.

- If possible, ignition sources should be avoided in an oxygen-enriched atmosphere; if used, they should be capsulated or have limited energy.

- Temperatures should be kept low, even under single-fault conditions, and must not exceed 300°C.

- Oxygen outlets must be at least 20 cm away from electrical socket outlets.

- Adequate ventilation should reduce the risk of developing an oxygen-enriched atmosphere.

6.4 Flammable Substances

There may be doubts about whether knowledge is power, but at least it is important to do things properly. This was demonstrated when a pupil tried to set his school on fire: In the cellar he poured out petrol, ignited a match, threw it onto the petrol, and ran away, without waiting to learn whether his plan worked. The burning match fell into the pool and was extinguished by the petrol, without causing any further harm.

The pupil did not realize that three requirements must be met in order to cause a fire:

1. A sufficient amount of **flammable material**

2. A sufficient, powerful **ignition source** to initiate the whole process

3.   A sufficient amount of **oxygen** to allow the chemical reaction to proceed

Because the pupil acted in a great hurry, there was not enough time to develop the necessary mixture of flammable gases with oxygen. In the end the plan failed, and the school still stands.

This example shows that because three requirements must be fulfilled to cause a fire, it is possible to avoid a fire if one of these requirements is not met.

Fire can occur only if three things are provided: flammable material, oxygen, and ignition energy!

Fire can be prevented if just one of these things is absent!

6.4.1 Characteristic Parameters

The danger of a flammable material can be characterized by three parameters:

1.   The **flash temperature** is the temperature above which flammable gas is developed from the liquid phase. For diethylether this temperature is –30°C, for petrol it is 0°C, and for alcohol +12°C. This means that even at room temperature these liquids develop flammable atmospheres without the need for additional energy.

2.   The **ignition temperature** indicates at what *surface temperatures* flammable atmospheres begin to burn. Diethylether at 170°C and benzene at 220°C prove to be especially

dangerous: A simple 100 W bulb with a surface temperature of 260°C can become a dangerous ignition source.

3. To ignite something, a **minimum ignition energy** is necessary. This is demonstrated in a campfire: Because the ignition energy of a match is too low to set a big branch on fire, a camper uses a step-by-step approach by preparing different layers and making sure that oxygen supply will be assured. With the limited ignition energy of a match, he first sets paper on fire, which in turn allows the smaller wooden pieces to start to burn, thus producing enough energy to finally light the larger branches.

Taking into account that the energy of electrostatic spark discharges from persons can be as high as 10,000 μJ (microjoules), substances such as diethylether, with a minimum ignition energy of 190 μJ, or internal body gases such as methane, with an ignition energy of 280 μJ, must be considered dangerous. By comparison, wood requires an ignition energy of 20,000 μJ.

6.4.2 Risk Zones

The operation theatre is one of the most sensitive parts of a hospital because it is one of the most dangerous places in regard to fire and explosion hazards. On the one hand, disinfectants and anaesthetic substances belong to dangerous flammable substances. On the other hand, oxygen and nitrous oxide are used, which are known to considerably reduce the minimum ignition energy down to 1 percent and make burns much easier, faster, and hotter. Finally, sufficient ignition energy is present, either because of the application of methods such as high frequency surgery or thermocautery or because of electrostatic spark discharges from persons to grounded objects.

These circumstances make it necessary to prevent explosion by a number of preventive measures: The first is to characterize zones in which explosive atmospheres might be encountered and that require special precautions. Two different zones can be distinguished in medically used rooms:

1.   **Zone G** comprises regions where flammable mixtures with *oxygen* can be expected. This might be within the gas pathways of an anaesthetic device, including the respiratory system of the patient, or its surroundings up to a distance of 5 cm from those parts where in normal conditions (e.g., leakage) or in single-fault conditions (e.g., breakage of a glass container) those mixtures can be expected.

2.   **Zone M** comprises those regions where flammable mixtures with *air* can be expected. This must be assumed to surround zone G, for instance, from 5 cm up to a distance of 25 cm from critical parts, such as glass containers. As anaesthetic gases and gases from disinfectants are heavier than air, they sink to the floor. For this reason the region below the operating table is also considered to be zone M. The dilution that increases until the mixture is too lean to be ignited is represented by the fact that zone M ends outside a pyramidal region, as shown in Figure 6.1.

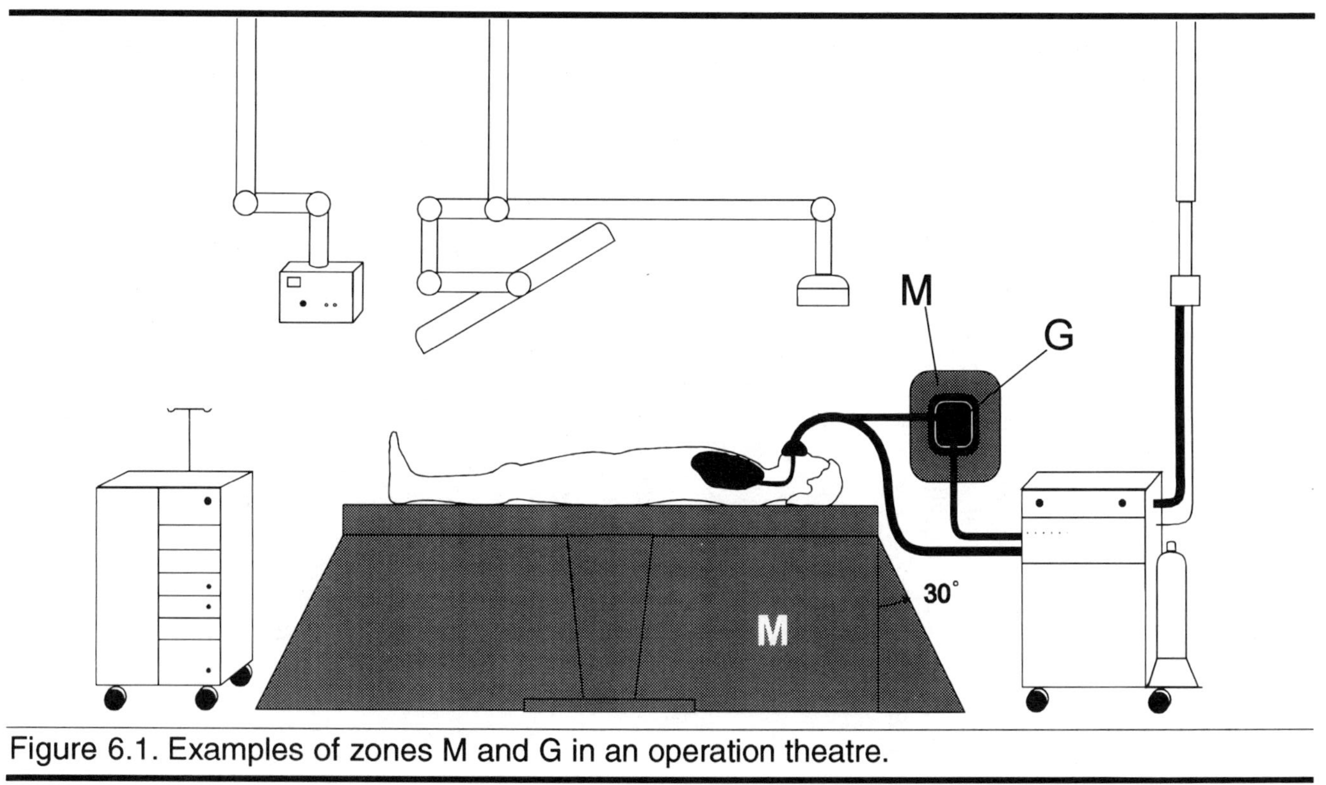

Figure 6.1. Examples of zones M and G in an operation theatre.

6.4.3 Safety Concept

The safety concept of avoiding explosion is based on three hierarchical steps: Avoiding explosive substances, avoiding possible ignition sources, and limiting possible harm.

Primary Explosion Protection

The most effective measure is to avoid an explosive atmosphere. This can be done by several approaches; first of all, if possible, by replacing dangerous substances with less dangerous ones. For example, extremely dangerous diethylether with an ignition temperature of only 170°C has been replaced by halogenic hydrocarbons like halothan, which has an almost fourfold higher ignition temperature of 635°C. Another means is preventing dangerous gas *concentrations* by enforced ventilation. Thus, Zone M can be neglected if the air in a room is replaced more than 15 times per hour by fresh air.

Device technology approaches comprise the reduction of leakage by improving the fit of an anaesthetic mask, which also improves the safety as well as the health of the medical staff. Another precaution is the use of nonflammable gases (inert gases) (e.g., nitrogen) to avoid any mixtures with oxygen, as has to be done during high frequency surgery at critical sites, such as the intestine or the larynx.

Secondary Explosion Protection

Secondary protection is designed to avoid *ignition* of an explosive atmosphere. This means excluding ignition sources that may be combined with the intended use of a device by using the explosion-protected device category AP or APG (see Figure 5.1) only in zones M and G. The strategy of explosion-protected device design includes capsulation of critical parts, such as the mains switch (with its switching spark), sufficient dimensioning of parts that may be under mechanical stress in case of an internal explosion, or limiting the energy of electric circuits. The latter works if the product of open-circuit voltage and short-circuit current does not exceed 10 VA. From this it follows that solely limiting voltage is not an adequate means of protection against explosions!

**Protective extra low voltage does not
by itself prevent explosions!**

Secondary explosion protection also includes the prevention of foreseeable accidental ignition sources, especially electrostatic spark discharges. Electrostatic charging is caused by friction or the separation of two materials with at least one being a poor conductor (see chapter 3). The most important strategy in preventing electrostatic discharging is to increase the electrical conductivity of chargeable objects. The conductivity of the floor can be increased by design or by the proper selection of material. It is common to have electrically conducting floors in operation theatres and intensive care units. However, it might turn out that this expensive investment does not lead to the expected results simply because insulating wax rather than the (more expensive) conducting wax has been used.

Electrostatic discharges are more probable in winter than in summer. Humid air, which dominates in the summer, promotes the early recombination of charges. Therefore, a further means to prevent electrostatic discharges is to keep air conductivity high by the use of air humidifiers. As an antistatic precaution, a relative humidity of 65 percent is considered to be sufficient.

In medical device technology the reduction of electrostatic charging can be avoided either by increasing the electrical conductivity of insulating parts that are subject to friction or by connecting insulated metallic parts with ground potential. Thus, anaesthetic or ventilation tube material contains carbon, and mobile devices and setups in an operation theatre should be connected to the floor by electrically conducting wheels.

Another means to avoid accidental ignition sparks is not to use extension mains cables, especially if the cable coupler is lying on the floor; in the case of an unintended stress, the plug can be pulled out of the socket, causing an interruption spark at the very region where the explosion hazard is relatively high.

Mains extension cables must not be used!

Finally, the prevention of accidental ignition requires avoiding surfaces or parts with temperatures above the flash temperature. This refers not only to thermocautery devices that need high temperatures, but also to objects with unintended surface heating, such as the bulbs in halogenic lamps. In the interior of medical electrical devices, there are parts that are allowed to reach high temperatures even in normal condition, such as power resistors, amplifiers, or poor electrical contacts. In single-fault conditions transformers are allowed to reach temperatures up to 210°C.

Tertiary Explosion Protection

The replacement of dangerous substances and the avoidance of ignition sources are very important. These measures should, however, be assisted by employing the principle of keeping the *consequences* of an explosion *as small as possible*. This applies to all situations, in an operation theatre as well as in a laboratory. This requires that amounts of dangerous substances be kept as small as possible, for instance, by taking from a storage vessel only the amount that is immediately needed, not the amount for the whole working day. In regard to device technology, tertiary explosion protection can be achieved by restricting possible damage to a predetermined region (e.g., by capsulation of critical parts by a pressure-releasing ductile cover).

7 Electric Power Supply

When medical staff are asked the meaning of differently colored mains socket outlets in an operation theatre, the reaction is typical for most hospitals: They shrug their shoulders and reply, "It reflects the wish of the architect". With this response they unintentionally prove themselves to be risk factors: All medical staff must know which socket outlet should be supplied with current under every circumstance. This knowledge allows one to operate life-supporting devices, even in power supply failure situations. In addition, it is important to know that there are mains socket outlets belonging to different electric circuits and which mains socket outlets belong to which circuits. This allows one to equally distribute the electric load, and to avoid power supply interruption due to overload and the simultaneous failure of several electromedical devices. At a minimum it is important to know which mains socket outlets are still fed after the circuit breaker has been activated in order to connect life-supporting devices to these outlets.

This chapter will show how the availability of electric power is assured in hospitals in case of the accidental interruption of normal power supply, as well as in single-fault and overload conditions.

7.1 The Need for Electric Power

The requirements for electric power supply within hospitals differ from those in a household situation: There is a need for increased protection against electric shock. In addition, as electricity is necessary to operate life-supporting systems, there is a need for increased reliability of the power supply in the event of a power supply failure and in a single-fault condition.

Economically, it is not feasible to provide expensive installation systems throughout the hospital similar to those needed in the most critical location, the operation theatre. Therefore, according to their demands on the electric installation system, medically used rooms are divided into three groups (IEC 64-629:1992):

1. **Group 0** rooms are those where *electric installation does not play any special role* in regard to safety. This might be because there is no intended use of medical electrical devices, because class II medical electrical devices are used, or because the devices have an internal power supply only, or because they have no applied parts at all. Examples are operating wash rooms, operating sterilization rooms, central monitoring rooms, and so on.

2. **Group 1** rooms are locations where *some emergency power supply* is needed, but where *interruption* of medical electrical device application *can be accepted* in single-fault situations. In such rooms surgically invasive treatments might be performed, but interruption of the use of medical electrical devices would not pose harm to the patient. Examples are rooms for general examination and treatment, electrophysiologic diagnosis, endoscopy, general radiologic diagnosis,

nuclear medicine, magnetic resonance, haemodialysis, and so on.

3. **Group 2** comprises the most critical locations where life-supporting devices might be used and where large surgical operations might be performed, including on the heart. These uses require the highest demands on the power supply system: It is not only necessary to provide electric power during a power supply failure (e.g., following a direct lightning discharge [*supply reliability*]). If a heart-lung machine failed because the installation fuse has been blown in a single-fault situation of a protectively earthed device, the physician might be protected, but the patient would be at risk. There is a need for a *fail-safe supply* power feeding system.

7.2 Additional Safety Means

Enhanced protection against electric shock, which has already been addressed in chapter 4, implies that protection means must assure that even in a single-fault condition no voltage is accessible that is larger than the MSELVs of 25 V (alternating current) or 60 V (direct current), which are equal to half the values permitted in daily life.

7.2.1 Residual Current Protective Device

Electrical installations for medical rooms should be provided with an additional means of protection. As already mentioned in chapter 4, energy supplies generally have one pole connected to the ground (grounded power systems). This makes it necessary to insulate all live parts carefully from earthed parts because each could be a counterpole for a (short) circuit. If insulation fails, a part of the total current prematurely flows to the ground; in this case, at the distribution box forward and backward current flow is unequal. This very fact, however, can be used for an additional protection means in group 0 and group 1 locations: *Residual current protective devices* are used to monitor the sum of forward and backward currents continuously and to interrupt the circuit in case of an insulation failure-induced current imbalance. Within hospitals residual current protective devices should be activated at failure currents of only **30 mA,** far below the level for the activation of overcurrent protection devices at the distribution box that are set into action by currents over tens of amperes!

This not only gives evidence of the failure but also ends the failure situation by interrupting the relevant electric circuit. It is just this undisputed advantage that in an operation theatre affects the reliability of the power supply and may lead to danger to the patient. In a single-fault situation not only is one device affected; all devices connected to the same electric circuit are affected. However, a means of protection that indirectly poses risk to the patient cannot be accepted.

A solution to this dilemma that allows one to meet both requirements—double protection and energy supply reliability—is given by an (expensive) principle previously mentioned: the use of insulated power supply systems with all live parts insulated from the earth. If a short circuit occurs to grounded parts, nothing happens! This is because the electric (failure) circuit remains open; the only thing that occurs is that the insulated power supply system changes to a grounded system—something which already applies to the rest of the hospital. Only on a second independent failure, affecting the counterpole, will something occur at any other locations as well (e.g., a short circuit blowing the installation fuse and interrupting the electric circuit [Figure 7.1]).

Of course, the additional safety of an insulated power supply system increases cost; in this case, additional expense results from the installation of an extra safety transformer that must be large enough to supply the necessary power. In most cases the transformer is located in the electric distribution box that feeds the operation theatre.

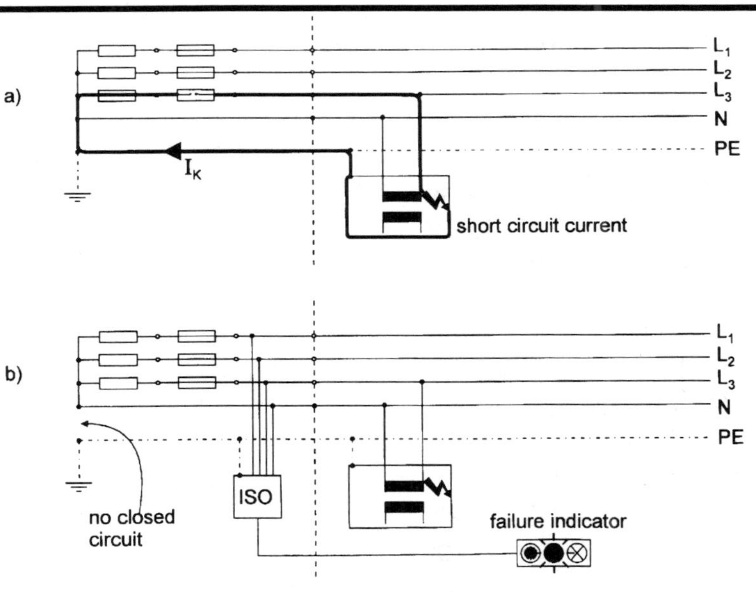

Figure 7.1. Consequences of an insulation failure in an earthed and insulated power supply system.

7.2.2 Insulation Monitoring Device

Insulated power supply systems exhibit a disadvantage: They do *not* allow one to become aware of a single insulation failure. Therefore, such failures would remain undetected until they were identified at the next safety inspection or until a second failure occurred. Since safety means that interrupt an electric circuit (such as a residual current protective device) would not solve the problem, another safety means must be chosen: an insulation monitoring device that continuously monitors the insulation resistance between all live parts and the earth potential. If an insulation failure occurs, there is still no reason for panic; the failure is indicated optically and acoustically (the acoustic alarm can be prompted only), and the surgical team can proceed with its work. At the end of treatment, the failure can be located and eliminated without any stress.

Fortunately, single faults are rare events. This, however, makes it necessary to check the proper functioning of the insulation monitoring device by regularly pressing the available test button. By this, a failure is simulated by the internal connection of a live part with the ground via a test resistance. The regular (e.g., monthly) check by the user (!) not only allows one to test the proper function of the acoustical alarm but also the functioning of the green (normal) operation indicator lamp and the red (failure) indicator lamp. Because this check affects neither the power supply nor the electrical installation, there is no reason not to perform it, even at short time intervals.

**Insulation monitoring devices must be checked
regularly by the medical staff!**

7.3 Emergency Power Supply

We know that because of thunderstorms, environmental disasters, wars, or major technical failures (e.g., in transformer stations), long-term feeding interruptions can occur. In general, besides some discomfort, there is little consequence in households. (They could, however, lead to increases in the birth rate, as could be observed after the extended power supply interruption in New York.) A long-term interruption in hospitals cannot be accepted, because they must to be able to provide at least some emergency service continuously.

The requirement of supply reliability is assured by providing two different independent additional voltage sources: One is a slowly available, **safety power supply source** with a changeover time **up to 15 seconds,** commonly a centrally located diesel generator. It must be able to maintain the power supply for at least 24 hours, and is intended to feed electromedical equipment in Group 2 rooms, the medical gas supply system, safety lighting, safety services, selected lifts, the ventilation system, the paging system, and so on.

In addition, a rapidly available, **additional power supply source** with a changeover time up to **0.5 seconds,** commonly decentralized sets of batteries, should be available for selected appliances, such as operating table luminaires.

The safety power supply system and the additional power supply system allow the continuous operation of the most important equipment, provided their electrical circuits are not overloaded. The greatest risk occurs during the changeover period. Therefore, automatic supply transfer is activated with different time delays, according to the different priorities of electrical appliances. So, for instance, it is acceptable for emergency lighting in a hall to be off for some seconds; during a critical phase of a surgical operation, however, a similar period of darkness in an operation theatre could endanger the patient.

In locations where not all the available socket outlets are connected to emergency power supply circuits, such as in a surgical ambulance, it is important to be able to identify the emergency power supply socket outlets reliably. In general, this is not yet standardized. Inscriptions or colour codes (e.g., green for socket outlets with changeover time up to 15 seconds and orange for changeover times up to 0.5 seconds) can be used; however, the medical staff must know the meaning and consequences of the marking. Life-supporting devices must be connected to the adequate socket outlet!

**Additional power supply socket outlets
must be known!**

7.4 Overload

Insulated power supply systems improve power supply reliability but cannot prevent the accidental interruption of electric circuits. This occurs if too many devices are connected to the same electric circuit, and the installation circuit breaker is activated by overload. A risk factor for this event is the use of flexible multiple socket outlets (see chapter 4). To reduce the risk for patients, at each patient's place of treatment, at least two socket outlets must be installed that are connected to different electric circuits. This should allow the provision of active feeding points for life-supporting devices even if one electric circuit is interrupted.

When seeking to avoid overload conditions, the electrical **load** must be equally distributed among the available electric circuits rather than the socket outlets! It is not the pure number of devices that is important, but the power consumption of the devices. This is usually indicated on the type label, in most cases at the rear of a device (see chapter 5).

While allocating devices to different socket outlets, well-trained staff are aware of the different emergency power supply facilities. Therefore, they differentiate between life-supporting and uncritical devices.

To allow the proper connection of medical electrical devices to socket outlets, it is necessary to have the socket outlets marked with the number of their electric circuit, to check that number, and to know what to do in case of an overload circuit interruption.

With respect to their power consumption, electrical devices should be equally allocated to the available electrical circuits!

Literature

Bergveld, P. 1978. *Elektromedizinische Gerätekunde.* Stuttgart: Thieme Verlag.

Biegelmeier, G. 1986. *Wirkungen des elektrischen Stromes auf Menschen und Nutztiere.* Berlin: VDE-Verlag.

Brinkmann, S. H. 1982. *Der Elektrounfall.* Berlin: Springer-Verlag.

Dalziel, C. F. 1961. The Threshold of Perception Currents. *AIEEE Transactions* 73:990–996.

Flamm, H., ed. 1994. *Angewandte Hygiene in Krankenhaus und Arztpraxis.* Wien: Dieter Göschl Verlag.

Fleming, D. G., and B. N. Feinberg, eds. 1976. *Handbook of Engineering in Medicine and Biology.* Cleveland: CRC Press, Inc.

Gärtner, A. 1992. *Sicherheit im Alltag der Medizintechnik.* Köln: Verlag TÜV Rheinland.

Haase, H. 1972. *Statische Elektrizität als Gefahr.* Weinheim: Verlag Chemie.

Harder, H. J. 1965. *Explosionsschutz.* Berlin: Springer-Verlag.

Harder, H. J. 1965. *Technische Sicherheitsprobleme im Operationstrakt.* Berlin: Springer-Verlag.

Hofheinz, W. 1991. *Schutztechnik mit Isolationsüberwachung.* Berlin: VDE-Verlag.

Hörmann, W., and A. Haslinger. 1992. *Rechtskunde für Gesundheitsberufe.* Wien: Dieter Göschl Verlag.

Hutten, H. ed. 1990. *Biomedizinische Technik,* vol. 1–4. Berlin: Springer-Verlag.

Koren, H. 1974. *Environmental Health and Safety.* New York: Pergamon.

Krasselt, J. M., and R. Flechsig. 1990. *Sauerstoff im Krankenhaus.* Köln: Verlag TÜV Rheinland.

Kuhlmann, A. 1981. *Einführung in die Sicherheitswissenschaft.* Wiesbaden: Viehweg Verlag.

Kupfer, J. 1987. *Elektrischer Strom als Unfallursache.* Berlin: Verlag Tribüne.

Leitgeb, N. 1990. *Strahlen, Wellen, Felder.* München: DTV Verlag; Stuttgart: Thieme Verlag.

Leitgeb, N. 1995. *Sicherheit in der Medizintechnik.* Renningen-Malmsheim: Expert Verlag.

Morse, H. N. 1986. *The Law and Medical Electronics: 50 Medical Malpractice Cases.* Available from Measurements & Data Corp., 2994 West Liberty Ave., Pittsburgh PA 15216.

Menke, W., ed. 1989. *Handbuch Medizintechnik.* Landsberg/Lech: Ecomed-Verlag. (updatable looseleaf booklet)

Perrow, C. 1984. *Normal Accidents: Living with High Risk Technologies.* New York: Basic Books.

Sam, U. 1969. *Neue Ergebnisse über die elektrische Gefährdung des Menschen bei Teildurchströmungen.* Hannover: VDRI-Jahrbuch.

Schmatz, H., and M. Nöthliches. 1987. *Sicherheitstechnik.* Berlin: Erich Schmidt Verlag. (updatable looseleaf booklet)

Skiba, R. 1985. *Taschenbuch der Arbeitssicherheit.* Berlin: Erich Schmidt Verlag.

Steuer, W. 1991. *Hygiene und Technik im Krankenhaus.* Ehningen: Expert Verlag.

Stoner, D. L., J. B. Smathers, W. A. Hyman, D. E. Clapp, and D. D. Duncan. 1982. *Engineering a Safe Hospital Environment.* New York: John Wiley & Sons.

Sudkamp, N. 1991. *Elektrische Anlagen im Krankenhaus.* Köln: Verlag TÜV Rheinland.

von der Mosel, H. A. 1992. *Medizintechnik für Pflegekräfte.* Melsungen: Bibliomed Verlag.

Webster, J. G. 1975. *Medical Instrumentation: Application and Design.* Boston: Houghton-Mifflin Co.

Index